Weight Loss Journal for Women

Mondo Nutrizionale

ISBN: 978-1-4717-2002-4

Hello! Ready to start this path?

Start by filling out your presentation form and taking measurements of your body to see from month to month how it will evolve!

After filling out the two forms, start your 90-day journey where you will have to write when, how and what you eat in the various sections, how much you drink/sleep, physical activity, your mood, and bad habits.

Every 15 days you will find a page to complete to write your improvements/ worsening, thus having the opportunity to see the progress of your path.

You can also follow a written path that will help you to stimulate your motivation to overcome every obstacle.

Just remember one thing! You must always be honest and do not be afraid of failing, you must go forward with commitment and dedication, only so you will achieve your goal!

That said, have a good start!

My presentation

Name: ....

Surname: ....

Date of birth: ....

Height: ....

Weight: ....

Build: ....

Diseases, intolerances, allergies:

....

Shape weight: ⟶ Objective:

☐ Underweight
☐ Normal weight
☐ Overweight

☐ Losing weight
☐ Being healthy
☐ Muscle development
☐ Weight gain

Do you do physical activity?   ☐ Yes ☐ No

Do you drink alcohol?   ☐ Yes ☐ No

Do you smoke?   ☐ Yes ☐ No

Write your goals

First goal

Motivate your goal

Second goal

Motivate your goal

Third goal

Motivate your goal

Shoot and paste your initial photo

Front

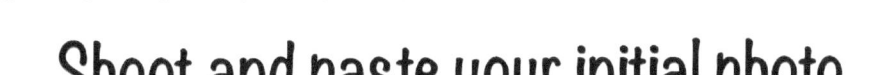

Shoot and paste your initial photo

Back

Ready to turn your life around?

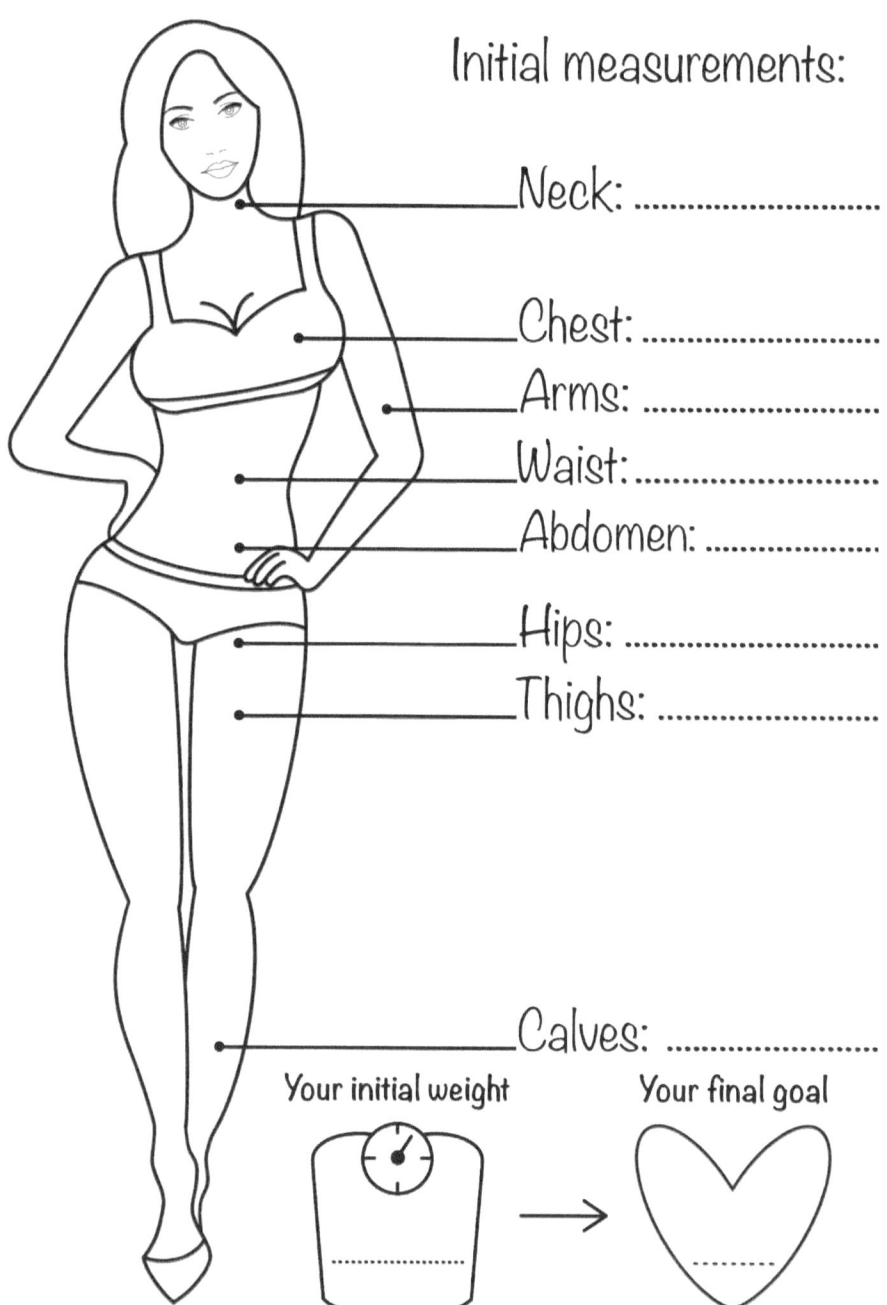

Initial measurements:

Neck: ....

Chest: ....
Arms: ....
Waist: ....
Abdomen: ....

Hips: ....
Thighs: ....

Calves: ....

Your initial weight

Your final goal

....

....

Mark your own path

During these 90 days mark with an "X" every day when you will complete this diary. Seeing as the sheet fills up will give you the right charge to not give up and finish your path!

First Month						
	1	2	3	4	5	6
	7	8	9	10	11	12
	13	14	(15)	16	17	18
	19	20	21	22	23	24
	25	26	27	28	29	(30)

Second Month						
	31	32	33	34	35	36
	37	38	39	40	41	42
	43	44	(45)	46	47	48
	49	50	51	52	53	54
	55	56	57	58	59	(60)

Third Month						
	61	62	63	64	65	66
	67	68	69	70	71	72
	73	74	(75)	76	77	78
	79	80	81	82	83	84
	85	86	87	88	89	(90)

Week 1

The word diet has taken on a negative meaning characterized by renunciations, strict rules, and temporary remedies in view of the summer or following the holidays but, in reality, the etymology of the term does not allude to any of this. Once, in fact, following a diet meant respecting the rules that taught **every aspect** of everyday life, to have a constant care of one's life in every nuance, from nutrition to physical exercise, to rest.

The task of this food diary is to accompany you in a 13-week journey of challenges and obstacles (otherwise what path would it be?) in which you will learn to have more awareness in the choices you make every day and to correct your habits, just as it was done in ancient times, in such a way as to constantly take care of you and dispel those myths that you have always considered absolute truth because of the beliefs that have forged you.

A food diary is useful because it keeps track of everything we eat and makes us aware of our mistakes: without a report, in fact, it is very difficult to have a realistic view of what we actually eat, especially if during meals we do something else and we are not fully present, but we will talk about this next week.

It is important to understand that compiling the food diary is not just about passively writing down a list of all the foods we have consumed during the week: it is about bringing awareness into our lives and, to do this, we also need to pay attention to the emotions we feel during meals.

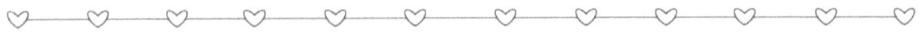

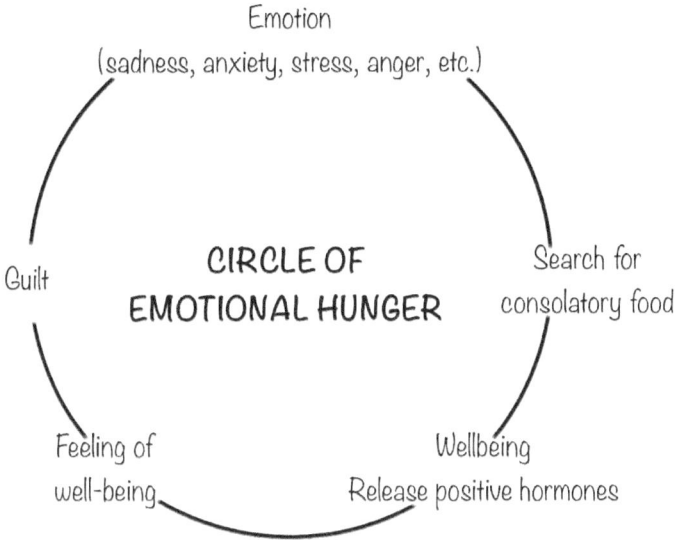

How many times have you had your stomach stuffed with nerves or finished a bowl of ice cream without realizing it in front of a movie or to drown our sadness?

The food diary also serves to keep track of the feelings we feel before, during and after the meal, to understand how many times we eat with the mind and how many times, instead, we let ourselves be guided by our body.

Having written all this in black and white, we will have a general picture of our relationship with food, our habits and we will be more motivated to vary or try something new.

Challenge of the week:
FILL OUT THE DIARY AT THE END OF EACH MEAL, FOCUSING YOUR ATTENTION ON THE EMOTIONS YOU FELT BEFORE, AFTER AND DURING.

Days ♡ | Date ....../ ....../ ......

♡ ♡ ♡ ♡ ♡ ♡ ♡ ♡ ♡ ♡

Breakfast   Lunch   Dinner

Snack I   Snack 2   Water

Sleep

Kcal

What time did you eat?

Breakfas: .... Lunch: .... Dinner: .... Snack I: .... Snack 2: ....

Supplements/ ....   ♡   Sports activities

Bad habits: How do you feel today?
Cigarettes
Alcohol   ☺ ☹ ☺ ☹ ☺
Sweets
Coffee   Other: ....

Notes of the day

♡ ♡ ♡ ♡ ♡ ♡ ♡ ♡ ♡ ♡

Days ♡②   Date ....../ ....../ ......

Breakfast   Lunch   Dinner

_____

Snack I   Snack 2   ☐ Water

                                      ☐ Sleep

                                      ☐ Kcal

What time did you eat?

Breakfas: .... Lunch: .... Dinner: .... Snack I: .... Snack 2: ....

Supplements/ ....   ♡ Sports activities

Bad habits: How do you feel today?
Cigarettes
Alcohol   ☺ ☹ 😐 😠 😴
Sweets
Coffee   Other: ....

Notes of the day

Days ♡ 3   Date ....../ ....../ ......

Breakfast   Lunch   Dinner

Snack 1   Snack 2   ⬜ Water

▢ Sleep

🍽 Kcal

What time did you eat?

Breakfas: ....   Lunch: ....   Dinner: ....   Snack 1: ....   Snack 2: ....

Supplements/ ....   ♡ Sports activities

Bad habits: How do you feel today?
Cigarettes
Alcohol   ☺ ☹ 😐 😠 😴
Sweets
Coffee   Other: ....

Notes of the day

Days ♡4 Date ....../ ....../ ......

Breakfast   Lunch   Dinner

Snack 1   Snack 2   🥛 Water

🛏 Sleep

🍽 Kcal

What time did you eat?

Breakfas: .... Lunch: .... Dinner: .... Snack 1: .... Snack 2: ....

Supplements/ ....   Sports activities

Bad habits: How do you feel today?
Cigarettes
Alcohol   ☺   ☹   😐   😠   😴
Sweets
Coffee   Other: ....

Notes of the day

Days ♡5♡   Date ....../ ....../ ......

Breakfast   Lunch   Dinner

Snack 1   Snack 2

♡ Water

♡ Sleep

♡ Kcal

What time did you eat?

Breakfas: ....   Lunch: ....   Dinner: ....   Snack 1: ....   Snack 2: ....

Supplements/ ....   ♡   Sports activities

Bad habits: ♡   How do you feel today?
Cigarettes
Alcohol   ☺   ☹   😐   😠   😴
Sweets
Coffee   Other: ....

Notes of the day

Days 6

Date ....../ ....../ ......

Breakfast

Lunch

Dinner

Snack 1

Snack 2

Water

Sleep

Kcal

What time did you eat?

Breakfas: .... Lunch: .... Dinner: .... Snack 1: .... Snack 2: ....

Supplements/ ....

Sports activities

Bad habits:
Cigarettes
Alcohol
Sweets
Coffee

How do you feel today?

Other: ....

Notes of the day

Days ♡ 7   Date ....../ ....../ ......

Breakfast   Lunch   Dinner

_____   _____   _____
_____   _____   _____
_____   _____   _____

Snack 1   Snack 2   🥛 Water

_____   _____   🛏 Sleep

_____   _____   🍽 Kcal

What time did you eat?

Breakfas: .... Lunch: .... Dinner: .... Snack 1: .... Snack 2: ....

Supplements/ ....   ♡ Sports activities

Bad habits: ♡ How do you feel today?
Cigarettes
Alcohol   🙂 🙁 😐 😠 😴
Sweets
Coffee   Other: ....

Notes of the day

_____

Week 2

Last week I left you with a flea in your ear that hinted at **eating with our mind or letting us be guided by our bodies**, a sentence not too clear but now I'll explain.

If you think about it, most of the time it is our mind that directs our relationship with food, which, by now, has become anything but a matter of survival: Try to think about how many stakes you set for yourself or how many times you can't resist something you'd like to eat to death.

Thanks to mindful eating we can change perspective and educate ourselves to eat listening to our body through the feeling of satiety or hunger. Mindful eating does not follow strict rules, but it helps us to reach a state of psycho-physical balance that will allow us to be comfortable with ourselves, learning to listen to our body that knows perfectly how to regulate itself. The focal point of mindful eating is the **way** we eat, not what we eat.

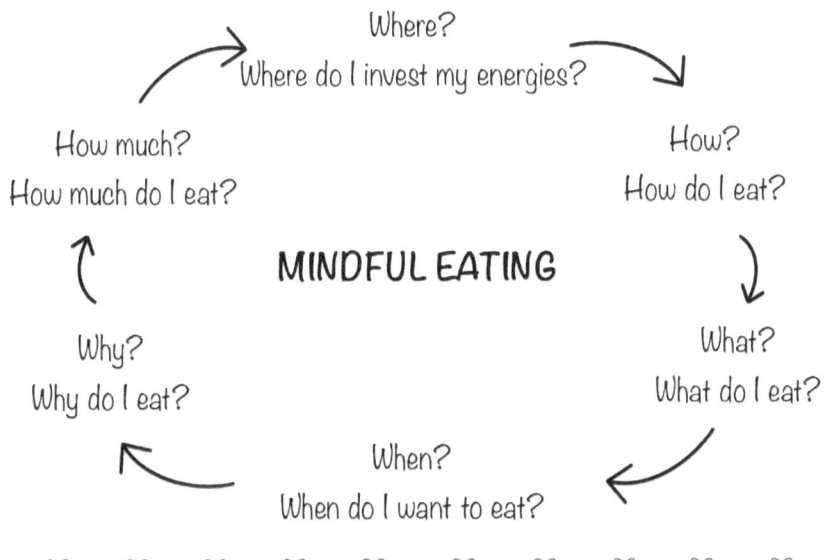

Where?
Where do I invest my energies?

How much?
How much do I eat?

How?
How do I eat?

MINDFUL EATING

Why?
Why do I eat?

What?
What do I eat?

When?
When do I want to eat?

This means avoiding to finish all the food we have in the dish if we are full, despite they have taught us to make an effort to do so; it means to reintroduce the foods of which we have been deprived and not to deny to do so because we are convinced that that given food **makes us fat**; means being present mentally both when we cook and while we eat, without distractions that do not make us enjoy the meal.

The focus of this week is awareness directed to nutrition and the phrases that we address to ourselves: for example, continuing to repeat to yourself sentences like "**I have to lose weight, otherwise I will never get into those pants/that dress**" and weighing yourself daily on the scale are two deleterious attitudes, as they make us identify with a number (the size of the clothes and what we read on the scale) and our subconscious is going to think that we're going to lose something that he's going to go after, and we're going to end up in the "yoyo loop".

If, instead, we use words more kind to ourselves as release instead of losing, mentally we will have the feeling of wanting to seek and regain a balance that will be maintained over time.

Challenge of the week:

AS IN THE EXAMPLE, THIS WEEK YOU HAVE THE TASK OF PAYING MORE ATTENTION TO THE SENTENCES YOU ADDRESS TO YOURSELF AND, WHEN YOU REALIZE THAT YOU ARE TOO HARSH, WRITE DOWN SENTENCES ON A SHEET OF PAPER

you will realize that these unpleasant words follow a pattern that repeats itself

AND **TURN THEM INTO POSITIVE THOUGHTS**. AFTER THIS OPERATION, PRACTICE REPEATING THE POSITIVE PHRASES IN YOUR MIND, SO AS TO TRAIN YOUR SUBCONSCIOUS TO BE KINDER.

Days ♡ 8   Date ....../ ....../ ......

Breakfast   Lunch   Dinner

Snack 1   Snack 2   ▢ Water

▢ Sleep

🍽 Kcal

What time did you eat?

Breakfas: .... Lunch: .... Dinner: .... Snack 1: .... Snack 2: ....

Supplements/ ....   ♡ Sports activities

Bad habits: How do you feel today?
Cigarettes
Alcohol   :) :(:| :((zz)
Sweets
Coffee   Other: ....

Notes of the day

Days ♡ 9

Date ....../ ....../ ......

Breakfast   Lunch   Dinner

Snack 1   Snack 2

Water

Sleep

Kcal

What time did you eat?

Breakfas: .... Lunch: .... Dinner: .... Snack 1: .... Snack 2: ....

Supplements/ ....

Sports activities

Bad habits:
Cigarettes
Alcohol
Sweets
Coffee

How do you feel today?

☺   ☹   😐   😠   😴

Other: ....

Notes of the day

Days 10 Date ....../ ....../ ......

Breakfast   Lunch   Dinner

Snack 1   Snack 2   🥤 Water

🛏 Sleep

🍽 Kcal

What time did you eat?

Breakfas: .... Lunch: .... Dinner: .... Snack 1: .... Snack 2: ....

Supplements/ ....

Sports activities

Bad habits:
Cigarettes
Alcohol
Sweets
Coffee

How do you feel today?

🙂 🙁 😐 😣 😴

Other: ....

Notes of the day

Days 〔♡〕

Date ....../....../......

Breakfast   Lunch   Dinner

Snack 1   Snack 2

♡ Water

🛏 Sleep

🍽 Kcal

What time did you eat?

Breakfas: .... Lunch: .... Dinner: .... Snack 1: .... Snack 2: ....

Supplements/...........   Sports activities

Bad habits: How do you feel today?
Cigarettes
Alcohol   🙂 🙁 😐 😠 😴
Sweets
Coffee   Other: ....

Notes of the day

Days ♡12♡   Date ....../ ....../ ......

Breakfast	Lunch	Dinner

Snack 1	Snack 2	

🥛 Water

🛏 Sleep

🍽 Kcal

What time did you eat?

Breakfas: .... Lunch: .... Dinner: .... Snack 1: .... Snack 2: ....

Supplements/ ....

Sports activities

Bad habits:
Cigarettes
Alcohol
Sweets
Coffee

How do you feel today?

☺ ☹ 😐 😠 😴

Other: ....

Notes of the day

Days ♥ 13　　Date ..../......./.......

Breakfast　　Lunch　　Dinner

Snack 1　　Snack 2　　☐ Water

☐ Sleep

☐ Kcal

What time did you eat?

Breakfas: ....　Lunch: ....　Dinner: ....　Snack 1: ....　Snack 2: ....

Supplements/ ....　♥　Sports activities

Bad habits:　　How do you feel today?
Cigarettes
Alcohol　　☺ ☹ 😐 😠 😴
Sweets
Coffee　　Other: ....

Notes of the day

Days ♡14

Date ....../ ....../ ......

Breakfast   Lunch   Dinner

Snack 1   Snack 2

🥛 Water

🛏 Sleep

🍽 Kcal

What time did you eat?

Breakfas: .... Lunch: .... Dinner: .... Snack 1: .... Snack 2: ....

Supplements/ .... ♡ Sports activities

Bad habits:
Cigarettes
Alcohol
Sweets
Coffee

How do you feel today?

☺ ☹ 😐 😠 😴

Other: ....

Notes of the day

Week 3

This week we talk about portions: we throw the scales and learn to use our hands. The best way to educate ourselves to eat with our body and not with the mind is to adjust the portions intuitively, without the help of the scales but only listening to our hunger.

Think about it: do you really need to weigh all the food you eat?
If you do not have the slightest idea of the quantities, it is right to resort to the scale but, after a while cooking, you will be able to get the perfect portions for you by eye.

This does not mean abounding with doses or getting out of hand and, therefore, cooking too much: you can use tools that you usually use in the kitchen, such as glasses or spoons or you can think of using your hands directly.

- a portion of carbohydrates (pasta, bread, rice, potatoes) should be the size of a closed fist;

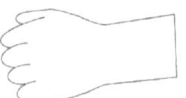

- one portion of fruit should be as large as two hands that make a cup - at least twice a day;

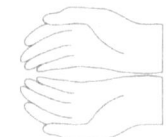

- a portion of good fat (extra virgin olive oil, sunflower oil, avocado, pistachios, almonds, hazelnuts) should be as large as the inch;

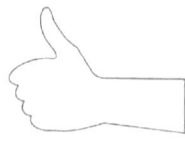

- a portion of protein (legumes, lean meat, fish, eggs) should be as large as the palm of your hand.

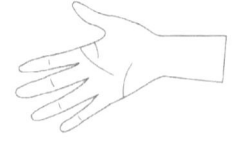

The only foods that can be ingested in large quantities are vegetables, while the rest must be managed with a unit of measurement to our liking and that we can get by reading the nutritional data on the back of the package, that always brings back to what a portion corresponds to

often it happens to eat too much dried fruit because it is considered a healthy food, and it is, but this does not mean that we must go for the entire package all at once.

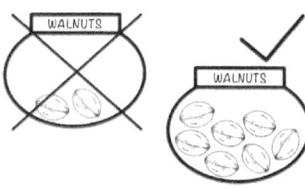

In addition, thanks to the food diary, we have the opportunity to record meals with constancy, so as to keep under control the calories we take compared to our daily needs.

Challenge of the week:

BEFORE YOU THROW THE KITCHEN SCALE IN THE TRASH, THIS WEEK TRY TO APPLY THE RULE OF PORTIONS FOR ONLY ONE MEAL BUT **EVERY DAY**: AT BREAKFAST, LUNCH, OR DINNER, AT YOUR DISCRETION.

Days ♡15♡   Date ....../ ....../ ......

Breakfast   Lunch   Dinner

Snack 1   Snack 2   🥛 Water

🛏 Sleep

🍽 Kcal

What time did you eat?

Breakfas: .... Lunch: .... Dinner: .... Snack 1: .... Snack 2: ....

Supplements/ ....

Sports activities

Bad habits:
Cigarettes
Alcohol
Sweets
Coffee

How do you feel today?

☺ ☹ 😐 😠 😴

Other: ....

Notes of the day

In these fifteen days

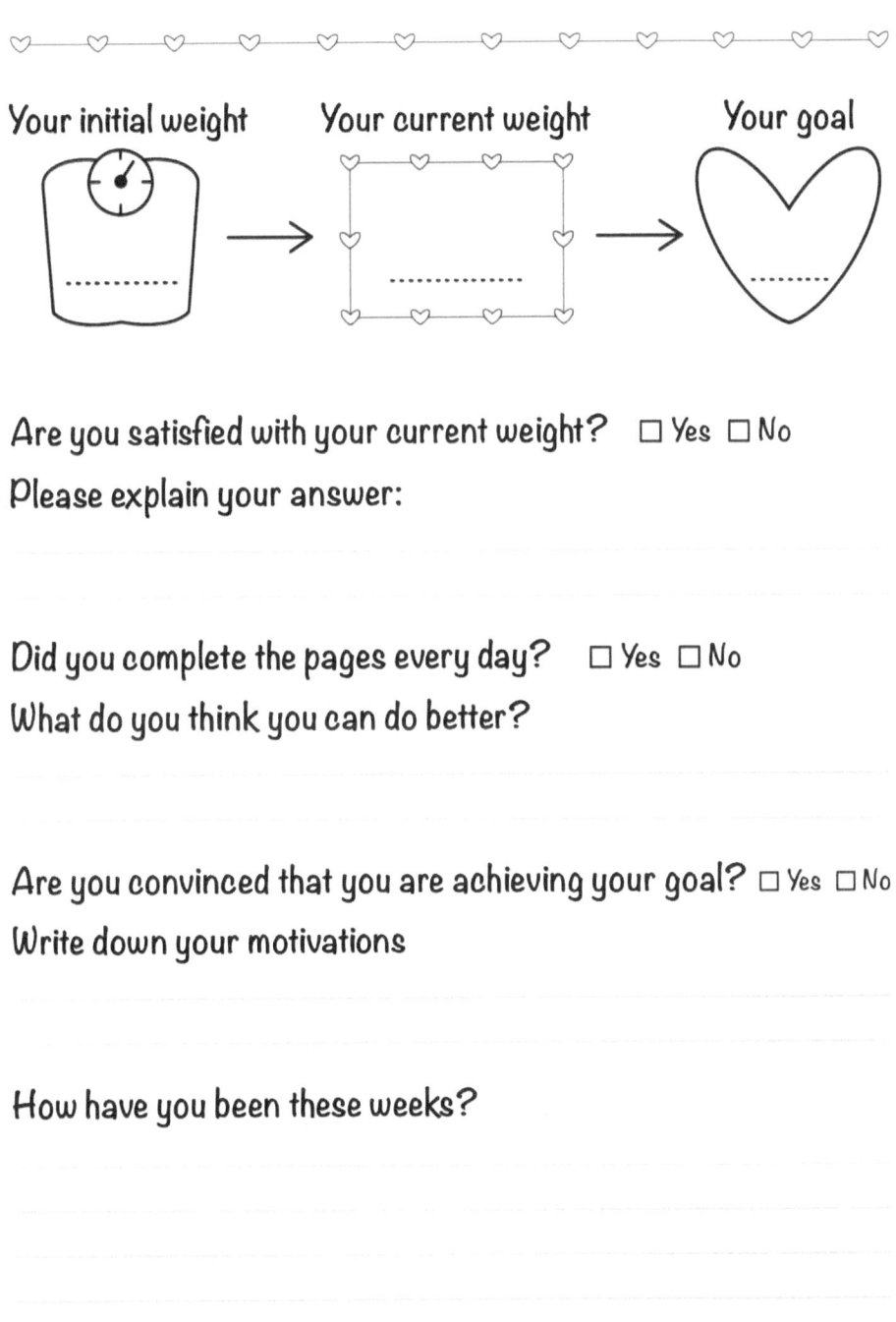

Your initial weight

Your current weight

Your goal

Are you satisfied with your current weight? ☐ Yes ☐ No

Please explain your answer:

Did you complete the pages every day? ☐ Yes ☐ No
What do you think you can do better?

Are you convinced that you are achieving your goal? ☐ Yes ☐ No
Write down your motivations

How have you been these weeks?

Days 〈16〉   Date ....../ ....../ ......

Breakfast   Lunch   Dinner

Snack 1   Snack 2   Water

Sleep

Kcal

What time did you eat?

Breakfas: .... Lunch: .... Dinner: .... Snack 1: .... Snack 2: ....

Supplements/ ....   Sports activities

Bad habits:
Cigarettes
Alcohol   How do you feel today?
Sweets
Coffee   Other: ....

Notes of the day

Days ♡ 17

Date ....../ ....../ ......

Breakfast

Lunch

Dinner

Snack 1

Snack 2

Water

Sleep

Kcal

What time did you eat?

Breakfas: .... Lunch: .... Dinner: .... Snack 1: .... Snack 2: ....

Supplements/ ....

Sports activities

Bad habits:
Cigarettes
Alcohol
Sweets
Coffee

How do you feel today?

☺ ☹ 😐 😣 😴

Other: ....

Notes of the day

Days ♡18♡   Date ....../ ....../ ......

Breakfast   ## Lunch   ## Dinner

_____   _____   _____
_____   _____   _____
_____   _____   _____

Snack 1   ## Snack 2   ♡ Water

_____   _____
                 _____   Sleep

                                        Kcal

What time did you eat?

Breakfas: .... Lunch: .... Dinner: .... Snack 1: .... Snack 2: ....

Supplements/ ....   ## Sports activities

Bad habits: ## How do you feel today?
Cigarettes
Alcohol   ☺ ☹ 😐 😠 😴
Sweets
Coffee   Other: ....

Notes of the day

Days 19   Date ....../ ....../ ......

Breakfast   ## Lunch   ## Dinner

Snack 1   ## Snack 2   Water

Sleep

Kcal

What time did you eat?

Breakfas: .... Lunch: .... Dinner: .... Snack 1: .... Snack 2: ....

Supplements/ ....   Sports activities

Bad habits: How do you feel today?
Cigarettes
Alcohol
Sweets
Coffee   Other: ....

Notes of the day

Days ♡20♡

Date ....../ ....../ ......

Breakfast	Lunch	Dinner

Snack 1   Snack 2

🥛 Water

🛏 Sleep

🍽 Kcal

What time did you eat?

Breakfas: .... Lunch: .... Dinner: .... Snack 1: .... Snack 2: ....

Supplements/ ....

Sports activities

Bad habits:
Cigarettes
Alcohol
Sweets
Coffee

How do you feel today?

☺ ☹ 😐 😠 😴

Other: ....

Notes of the day

Days ♡ 21   Date ....../ ....../ ......

Breakfast   Lunch   Dinner

_____   _____   _____
_____   _____   _____
_____   _____   _____

Snack 1   Snack 2   ▢ Water

_____   _____   ▢ Sleep

_____   _____   ▢ Kcal

What time did you eat?

Breakfas: .... Lunch: .... Dinner: .... Snack 1: .... Snack 2: ....

Supplements/ ....   ♡   Sports activities
                            │
                            ♡   _____
                            │
                            ♡
Bad habits: │   How do you feel today?
Cigarettes   ♡
Alcohol   │   ☺ ☹ 😐 😠 😴
Sweets   │
Coffee   ♡   Other: ....

Notes of the day _____

_____

Week 4

This week's keyword is a one-plate meal. The one-plate is a scheme that we can follow to compose each meal in a healthy way, and it is not a single course, as could be a salad or pizza.

Thanks to the one-plate we can eat in a healthy way because it is a complete and balanced meal: in fact, it provides our body with all the necessary nutrients such as carbohydrates, vitamins, lipids, proteins, minerals, and antioxidants in the right proportions.

The one-plate consists of a very simple formula:

50% carbohydrates from fruits and vegetables;
25% carbohydrates from whole grains or potatoes;
25% animal protein (meat, fish, and eggs) and vegetable protein (legumes).

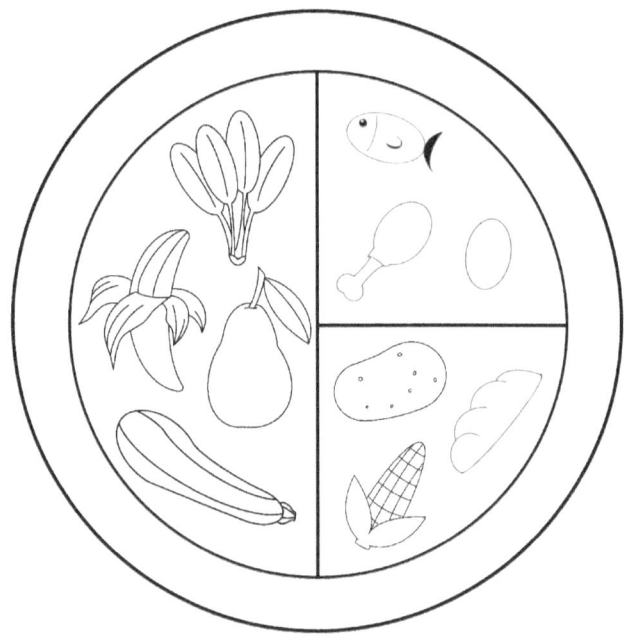

Vegetables, as we can see, are the protagonists of the one-plate, without considering the potatoes which, because of their starch content, are more similar to pasta.

To complete the one-plate, we must also take into account the good fats that we can use as condiments, such as extra virgin olive oil, dried fruit and oilseeds, not to mention the herbs and spices that, in addition to enriching the flavor of our dish, they bring many phytonutrients benefits to our body.

According to the above, the one-plate meals may be repetitive but it's the opposite! The more we play with the alternation between different types of food, the more our diet will be balanced, complete and varied also because the protein part cannot be composed only of meat or fish. Ideally you should consume fish more often (3 to 4 times a week), eggs, legumes, and white meat up to 3 times a week and, finally, red meat only once a week.

The same applies to carbohydrates in the form of potatoes or whole grains: we can alternate barley, spelt, rice and brown pasta.
Brown rice is a very versatile food: we can use it as a seasoning of stuffed vegetables or as a main course and is a valid alternative to pasta, as well as being an exceptional source of minerals and antioxidants.

Challenge of the week:
TRY TO COMPOSE THREE LUNCHES AND THREE DINNERS WITH DIFFERENT UNIQUE DISHES.

Days (22)　　Date ....../....../......

Breakfast　　Lunch　　Dinner

_____
_____
_____
_____

Snack 1　　Snack 2

Water

Sleep

Kcal

What time did you eat?

Breakfas: .... Lunch: .... Dinner: .... Snack 1: .... Snack 2: ....

Supplements/ ....　　Sports activities

Bad habits:　　How do you feel today?
Cigarettes
Alcohol　　:) :(:| :((zzz)
Sweets
Coffee　　Other: ....

Notes of the day

Days ♡23♡

Date ....../ ....../ ......

Breakfast

Lunch

Dinner

Snack 1

Snack 2

Water

Sleep

Kcal

What time did you eat?

Breakfas: .... Lunch: .... Dinner: .... Snack 1: .... Snack 2: ....

Supplements/ ....

Sports activities

Bad habits:
Cigarettes
Alcohol
Sweets
Coffee

How do you feel today?

Other: ....

Notes of the day

Days 24   Date ....../ ....../ ......

Breakfast   Lunch   Dinner

_____   _____   _____
_____   _____   _____
_____   _____   _____
_____   _____   _____

Snack 1   Snack 2   Water

_____   _____   Sleep

_____   _____   Kcal

What time did you eat?

Breakfas: .... Lunch: .... Dinner: .... Snack 1: .... Snack 2: ....

Supplements/ ....   Sports activities

Bad habits: How do you feel today?
Cigarettes
Alcohol   ☺ ☹ 😐 😠 😴
Sweets
Coffee   Other: ....

Notes of the day

Days 25   Date ....../ ....../ ......

Breakfast   Lunch   Dinner

Snack 1   Snack 2

 Water

 Sleep

 Kcal

What time did you eat?

Breakfas: .... Lunch: .... Dinner: .... Snack 1: .... Snack 2: ....

Supplements/............

Sports activities

Bad habits:
Cigarettes
Alcohol
Sweets
Coffee

How do you feel today?

Other: ....

Notes of the day

Days ♡26♡   Date ....../ ....../ ......

Breakfast   Lunch   Dinner

Snack 1   Snack 2   Water

                                  Sleep

                                  Kcal

What time did you eat?

Breakfas: .... Lunch: .... Dinner: .... Snack 1: .... Snack 2: ....

Supplements/ ....   Sports activities

Bad habits: How do you feel today?
Cigarettes
Alcohol   ☺ ☹ 😐 😠 😴
Sweets
Coffee   Other: ....

Notes of the day

Days ♡27♡

Date ....../ ....../ ......

Breakfast   Lunch   Dinner

Snack 1   Snack 2   🥤 Water

🛏 Sleep

🍽 Kcal

What time did you eat?

Breakfas: .... Lunch: .... Dinner: .... Snack 1: .... Snack 2: ....

Supplements/ ....   Sports activities

Bad habits: How do you feel today?
Cigarettes
Alcohol   ☺ ☹ 😐 😣 😴
Sweets
Coffee   Other: ....

Notes of the day

Days ♡28♡

Date ....../ ....../ ......

Breakfast

Lunch

Dinner

Snack 1

Snack 2

💧 Water

🛏 Sleep

🍽 Kcal

What time did you eat?

Breakfas: .... Lunch: .... Dinner: .... Snack 1: .... Snack 2: ....

Supplements/ ....

Sports activities

Bad habits:
Cigarettes
Alcohol
Sweets
Coffee

How do you feel today?

☺ ☹ 😐 😠 😴

Other: ....

Notes of the day

Week 5

From improving our skin, our vital functions and eliminating toxins, drinking more water is definitely a habit that each of us needs to adopt. But how many of us can drink the canons two liters every day? In case it's not clear, this week we're going to focus on this prodigious, colorless, tasteless chemical, which is the basis of ecosystems and all forms of life: water.

Our organism is composed mainly of water, and yet drinking at least two liters a day is the golden rule to feel good. For some it seems impossible, for other two liters are too few: the truth is that the amount of water to be consumed varies according to weight, the climate in which we live, the physical activity we practice and our state of health. Therefore, each of us needs to calculate how much water we need to drink according to our needs - a quick calculation that we can all do is to multiply 30ml of water per kg of body weight and then also consider the task and physical activity that we perform each day.

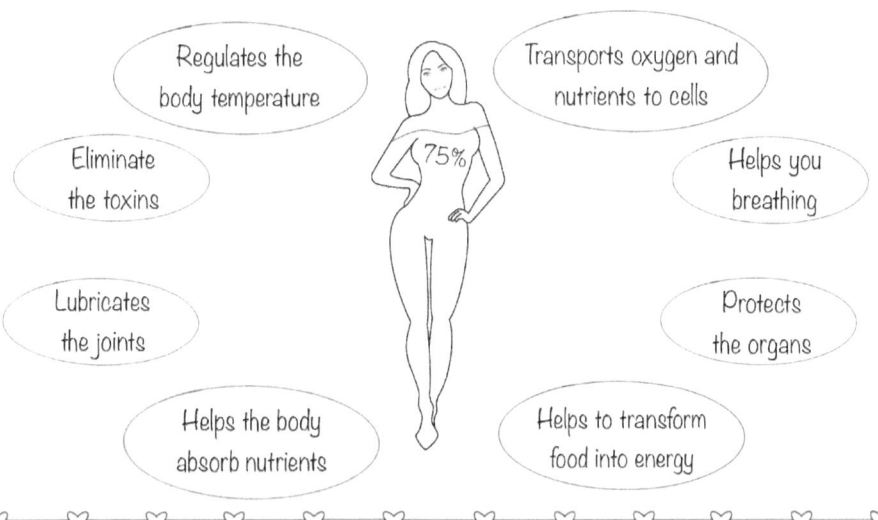

One mistake we all make is to drink more glasses of water all in one breath because, perhaps, at the end of the day we realized we had not drunk anything. This is a mistake because then our kidneys will have to work twice as hard. The ideal would be to have a bottle or a thermos always at hand (in fact, when the water is well in sight it is difficult not to remember to drink) and take a sip of water every 15 minutes, so as to stay hydrated constantly and adjust our metabolism.

If the taste of the water doesn't tell us anything, we can try the sparkling water that stimulates the receptors in our mouth and leave us that refreshing sensation, or we can try to create detox water by adding citrus fruits and a couple of slices of cucumbers, so it tastes better. Tea and herbal teas are not excluded from the amount of water to be consumed daily, so, in case a hot drink seems more comfortable than water at room temperature, we can fill a thermos and sip it throughout the day.

Another way to drink more water is to consume a good amount of fruits and vegetables - especially watermelons, strawberries, tomatoes, oranges, grapes, cherries, spinach and radishes are the most moisturizing foods.

In addition, there are several applications that can remind us to drink and that offer various tips for taking more water: we can try to rely on technology for a good cause!

Challenge of the week:

THIS WEEK YOU MUST FIND A WAY TO DRINK MORE, WHETHER IT'S TO CREATE DETOX WATER OR FILL A THERMOS OF YOUR FAVORITE HERBAL TEA, IF YOU'RE USED TO DRINKING ONLY DURING MEALS, STARTS TO CREATE SMALL DEVICES TO BE ABLE TO DRINK AT LEAST A LITER AND A HALF OF WATER EVERY DAY.

Days ♡ 29

Date ....../....../......

Breakfast　　Lunch　　Dinner

Snack 1　　Snack 2

♡ Water

♡ Sleep

♡ Kcal

What time did you eat?

Breakfas: ....　Lunch: ....　Dinner: ....　Snack 1: ....　Snack 2: ....

Supplements/............

Sports activities

Bad habits:
Cigarettes
Alcohol
Sweets
Coffee

How do you feel today?

☺ ☹ 😐 😣 😴

Other: ....

Notes of the day

Days 30   Date ....../ ....../ ......

Breakfast   Lunch   Dinner

Snack 1   Snack 2   Water

Sleep

Kcal

What time did you eat?

Breakfas: .... Lunch: .... Dinner: .... Snack 1: .... Snack 2: ....

Supplements/ ....   Sports activities

Bad habits: How do you feel today?
Cigarettes
Alcohol   :) :(:| >:(:o zzz
Sweets
Coffee   Other: ....

Notes of the day

How was your first month?

Let's get back in shape!

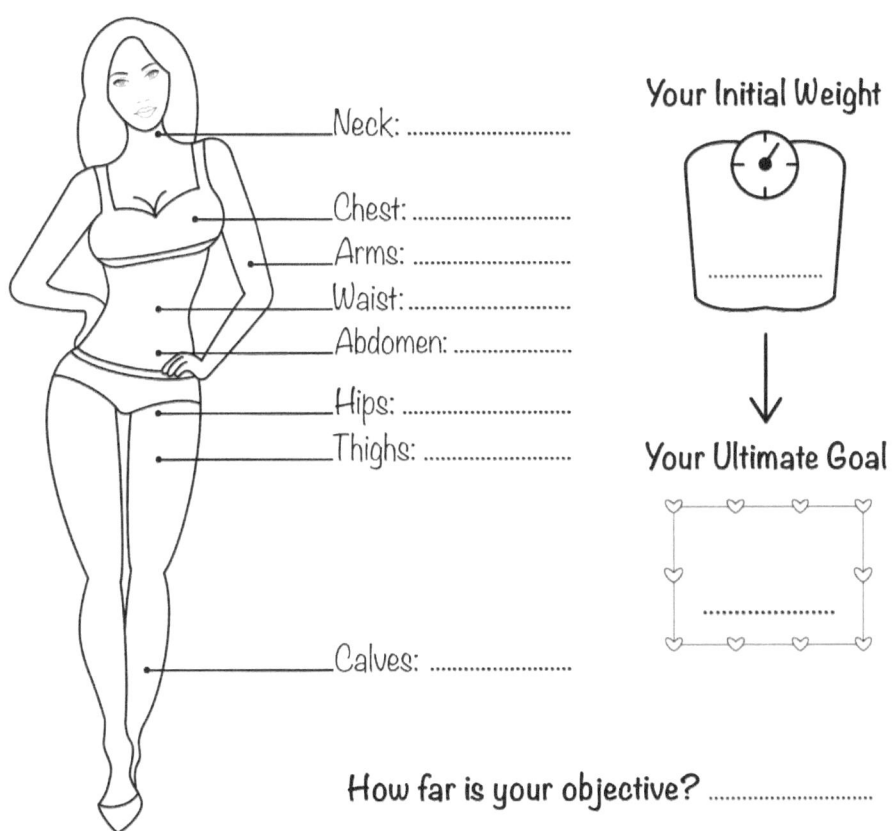

Neck: ....

Chest: ....

Arms: ....

Waist: ....

Abdomen: ....

Hips: ....

Thighs: ....

Calves: ....

Your Initial Weight

....

Your Ultimate Goal

....

How far is your objective? ....

Write your thoughts about these weeks!

Days 31   Date ....../....../......

Breakfast   Lunch   Dinner

Snack 1   Snack 2   Water

Sleep

Kcal

What time did you eat?

Breakfas: .... Lunch: .... Dinner: .... Snack 1: .... Snack 2: ....

Supplements/............   Sports activities

Bad habits: How do you feel today?
Cigarettes
Alcohol   :) :(:| >:(zzz
Sweets
Coffee   Other: ....

Notes of the day

Days ♥ 32   Date ....../ ....../ ......

Breakfast   Lunch   Dinner

Snack 1   Snack 2   Water

Sleep

Kcal

What time did you eat?

Breakfas: .... Lunch: .... Dinner: .... Snack 1: .... Snack 2: ....

Supplements/ ....   Sports activities

Bad habits: How do you feel today?
Cigarettes
Alcohol   ☺ ☹ 😐 😠 😴
Sweets
Coffee   Other: ....

Notes of the day

Days ♡33♡

Date ....../ ....../ ......

Breakfast

Lunch

Dinner

Snack 1

Snack 2

Water

Sleep

Kcal

What time did you eat?

Breakfas: .... Lunch: .... Dinner: .... Snack 1: .... Snack 2: ....

Supplements/ ....

Sports activities

Bad habits:
Cigarettes
Alcohol
Sweets
Coffee

How do you feel today?

☺ ☹ 😐 😠 😴

Other: ....

Notes of the day

Days ♥34♥

Date ....../ ....../ ......

Breakfast

Lunch

Dinner

Snack 1

Snack 2

Water

Sleep

Kcal

What time did you eat?

Breakfas: .... Lunch: .... Dinner: .... Snack 1: .... Snack 2: ....

Supplements/............

Sports activities

Bad habits:
Cigarettes
Alcohol
Sweets
Coffee

How do you feel today?

☺ ☹ 😐 😣 😴

Other: ....

Notes of the day

Days 35   Date ....../ ....../ ......

Breakfast   Lunch   Dinner

Snack 1   Snack 2   Water

Sleep

Kcal

What time did you eat?

Breakfas: .... Lunch: .... Dinner: .... Snack 1: .... Snack 2: ....

Supplements/ ....   Sports activities

Bad habits: How do you feel today?
Cigarettes
Alcohol
Sweets
Coffee   Other: ....

Notes of the day

Week 6

How many times are we stared horrified the word "fats" without knowing that they are not all harmful and there is a subdivision?

We cannot completely remove **fats** from our diet because they are an integral part of our vital functions. In fact, they are present in our cell and brain membranes, carry fat-soluble vitamins such as **A, D, E** and **K** and are a key element to keep our energy reserve alive.

As mentioned, fats are not all the same: some are good and useful to our body, while the bad ones, over time, involve risks and can lead to diseases such as diabetes, obesity, cancer, and cardiovascular diseases.

Saturated fats are not harmful if consumed in moderation and are in solid form at room temperature: mainly they are of animal origin such as whole milk, cheese, sour cream, butter, beef, and pork fat but can also be of vegetable origin such as tropical oils, such as coconut oil and palm oil.

Trans fats are the ones to avoid because they raise the level of cholesterol in the blood and are formed in the stomach of cattle and sheep or through hydrogenation, that is the process that converts a liquid oil into a solid fat.

Unsaturated fats, on the other hand, are good because they produce beneficial effects to our body and are divided into monounsaturated and polyunsaturated but must be taken in moderation because they are very caloric.

These include olive oil, avocado, walnuts, cashews, almonds, peanut butter (monounsaturated fats) but also flaxseed and some types of fish such as salmon, trout, mackerel, herring (polyunsaturated fats).

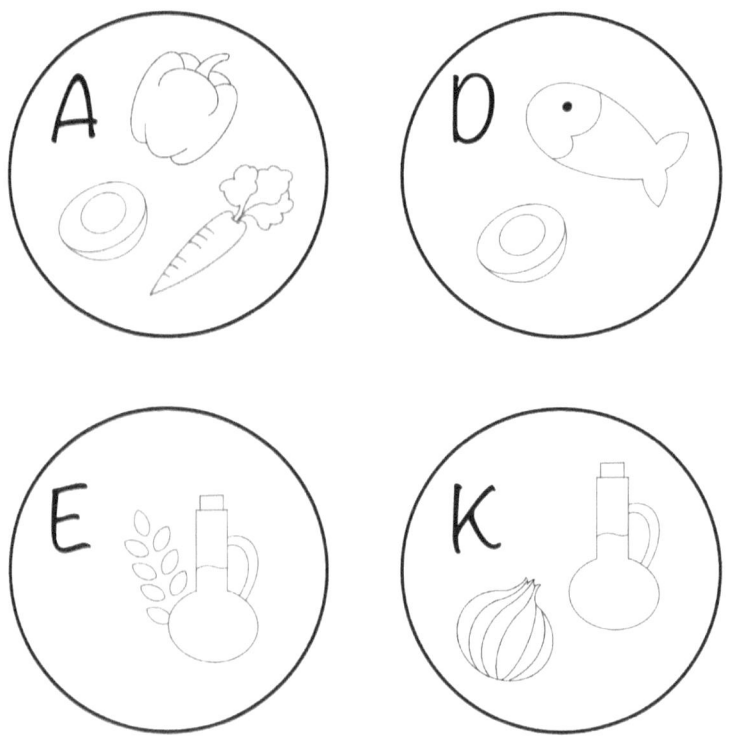

Challenge of the week:

DURING THE COURSE OF THIS WEEK, YOU WILL NEED TO SUPPLEMENT AN UNSATURATED FAT DURING ONE OF THE FIVE DAILY MEALS - FOR EXAMPLE: EATING ALMONDS AS A SNACK, PREPARING A SINGLE DISH THAT INCLUDES AVOCADO, HAVING BREAKFAST WITH PEANUT BUTTER...

Days ❤36 Date ....../ ....../ ......

Breakfast   ## Lunch   ## Dinner

Snack I   ## Snack 2

🥤 Water

😷 Sleep

🍽 Kcal

What time did you eat?

Breakfas: .... Lunch: .... Dinner: .... Snack I: .... Snack 2: ....

Supplements/ ....   Sports activities

Bad habits: How do you feel today?
Cigarettes
Alcohol   🙂 ☹️ 😐 😣 😴
Sweets
Coffee   Other: ....

Notes of the day

Days ♡37♡

Date ....../....../......

Breakfast   Lunch   Dinner

Snack 1   Snack 2

Water

Sleep

Kcal

What time did you eat?

Breakfas: .... Lunch: .... Dinner: .... Snack 1: .... Snack 2: ....

Supplements/ ....

Sports activities

Bad habits:
Cigarettes
Alcohol
Sweets
Coffee

How do you feel today?

☺ ☹ ☺ ☹ ☺

Other: ....

Notes of the day

Days 38   Date ....../ ....../ ......

Breakfast   Lunch   Dinner

Snack 1   Snack 2   🥛 Water

🛏 Sleep

🍽 Kcal

What time did you eat?

Breakfas: ....   Lunch: ....   Dinner: ....   Snack 1: ....   Snack 2: ....

Supplements/ ....   Sports activities

Bad habits: How do you feel today?
Cigarettes
Alcohol   🙂 🙁 😐 😠 😴
Sweets
Coffee   Other: ....

Notes of the day

Days ♡39♡

Date ....../ ....../ ......

Breakfast   Lunch   Dinner

Snack 1   Snack 2

🥛 Water

🛏 Sleep

🍽 Kcal

What time did you eat?

Breakfas: .... Lunch: .... Dinner: .... Snack 1: .... Snack 2: ....

Supplements/ ....

Sports activities

Bad habits:
Cigarettes
Alcohol
Sweets
Coffee

How do you feel today?

Other: ....

Notes of the day

Days 40   Date ....../ ....../ ......

Breakfast   Lunch   Dinner

Snack 1   Snack 2   Water

Sleep

Kcal

What time did you eat?

Breakfas: .... Lunch: .... Dinner: .... Snack 1: .... Snack 2: ....

Supplements/ ....   Sports activities

Bad habits: How do you feel today?
Cigarettes
Alcohol
Sweets   Other: ....
Coffee

Notes of the day

Days ♡41♡

Date ....../ ....../ ......

Breakfast

Lunch

Dinner

Snack 1

Snack 2

♡ Water

Sleep

Kcal

What time did you eat?

Breakfas: .... Lunch: .... Dinner: .... Snack 1: .... Snack 2: ....

Supplements/ ....

♡

Sports activities

Bad habits:
Cigarettes
Alcohol
Sweets
Coffee

How do you feel today?

☺ ☹ 😐 😣 😴

Other: ....

Notes of the day

Days 42   Date ....../ ....../ ......

Breakfast   Lunch   Dinner

Snack 1   Snack 2

Water

Sleep

Kcal

What time did you eat?

Breakfas: .... Lunch: .... Dinner: .... Snack 1: .... Snack 2: ....

Supplements/ ....   Sports activities

Bad habits: How do you feel today?
Cigarettes
Alcohol
Sweets
Coffee   Other: ....

Notes of the day

Week 7

This week, we're going to be fighting carbs, like we always have. Seriously, carbohydrates are seen as the enemies of well-being because they make us feel swollen but, in fact, they are part of a healthy and balanced diet. The only element to be eliminated in a diet, understood as a lifestyle and not in the most negative sense of the term, is excess.

Carbohydrates, in fact, are necessary to our body because they constitute our main source of energy and are absorbed in the form of glucose. Blood glucose levels, in turn, must remain constant so that we do not go into hypoglycemia or hyperglycemia, a condition that, in the long run, could lead to diabetes. So, when we are convinced that carbohydrates make you fat, we have not considered the amount we eat: carbohydrates make you fat when the excess glucose is deposited in the adipose tissue and, of course, turns into fat.

60% of the calories that we eat daily should come from carbohydrates and, among these, most should be taken from complex carbohydrates - in fact, carbohydrates are divided into simple (such as fructose and sucrose) and complex (like cereal starch) but what we have to base our diet on are carbohydrates that do not create glycemic changes of any kind, such as whole grains. Instead, the excess of refined flour, sugar, potatoes, refined rice, and white bread should be avoided.

Challenge of the week:

IF YOU ARE USED TO EATING A PLATE OF PASTA EVERY DAY, TRY TO VARY FOR AT LEAST THREE DAYS IN A ROW, BUYING WHOLE WHEAT PASTA AT THE SUPERMARKET OR OTHER TYPES OF CEREALS.

Days 43   Date ....../ ....../ ......

Breakfast   Lunch   Dinner

Snack 1   Snack 2   Water

Sleep

Kcal

What time did you eat?

Breakfas: ....   Lunch: ....   Dinner: ....   Snack 1: ....   Snack 2: ....

Supplements/ ....   Sports activities

Bad habits: How do you feel today?
Cigarettes
Alcohol   :) :(:| >:(zzz
Sweets
Coffee   Other: ....

Notes of the day

Days 44   Date ....../ ....../ ......

Breakfast   Lunch   Dinner

Snack 1   Snack 2   Water

Sleep

Kcal

What time did you eat?

Breakfas: .... Lunch: .... Dinner: .... Snack 1: .... Snack 2: ....

Supplements/ ....   Sports activities

Bad habits: How do you feel today?
Cigarettes
Alcohol   ☺ ☹ 😐 😠 😴
Sweets
Coffee   Other: ....

Notes of the day

Days 45

Date ....../ ....../ ......

Breakfast

Lunch

Dinner

Snack 1

Snack 2

🥤 Water

😷 Sleep

🍽️ Kcal

What time did you eat?

Breakfas: .... Lunch: .... Dinner: .... Snack 1: .... Snack 2: ....

Supplements/ ....

Sports activities

Bad habits:
Cigarettes
Alcohol
Sweets
Coffee

How do you feel today?

😊 🙁 😐 😖 😴

Other: ....

Notes of the day

In these forty-five days

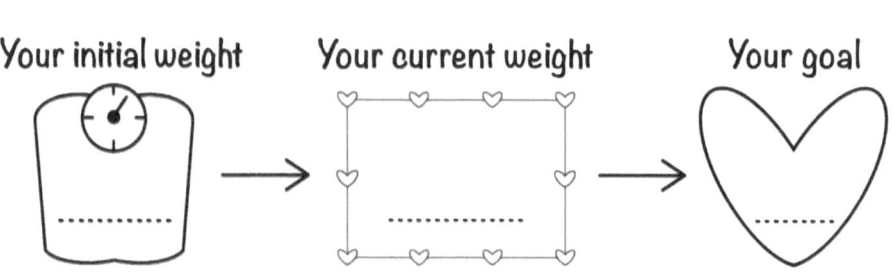

Your initial weight → **Your current weight** → **Your goal**

Are you satisfied with your current weight?   ☐ Yes ☐ No

Please explain your answer:

Did you complete the pages every day?   ☐ Yes ☐ No

What do you think you can do better?

Are you convinced that you are achieving your goal? ☐ Yes ☐ No

Write down your motivations

How have you been these weeks?

Days 46   Date ....../ ....../ ......

Breakfast   Lunch   Dinner

Snack 1   Snack 2   Water

Sleep

Kcal

What time did you eat?

Breakfas: .... Lunch: .... Dinner: .... Snack 1: .... Snack 2: ....

Supplements/ ....   Sports activities

Bad habits: How do you feel today?
Cigarettes
Alcohol   :) :(:| >:((zzz)
Sweets
Coffee   Other: ....

Notes of the day

Days ♡47♡　　Date ....../ ....../ ......

Breakfast　　Lunch　　Dinner

Snack 1　　Snack 2

🥛 Water

🛏 Sleep

🍽 Kcal

What time did you eat?

Breakfas: ....　Lunch: ....　Dinner: ....　Snack 1: ....　Snack 2: ....

Supplements/............　　Sports activities

Bad habits:　　How do you feel today?
Cigarettes
Alcohol
Sweets　　😊　😟　😐　😠　😴
Coffee

　　Other: ....

Notes of the day

Days 48

Date ..../......./.......

Breakfast

Lunch

Dinner

Snack 1

Snack 2

🥛 Water

🛏 Sleep

🍽 Kcal

What time did you eat?

Breakfas: .... Lunch: .... Dinner: .... Snack 1: .... Snack 2: ....

Supplements/............

Sports activities

Bad habits:
Cigarettes
Alcohol
Sweets
Coffee

How do you feel today?

🙂 🙁 😐 😠 😴

Other: ....

Notes of the day

Days ♡49♡

Date ....../ ....../ ......

Breakfast	Lunch	Dinner

Snack 1	Snack 2	
		🥛 Water
		🛏 Sleep
		🍽 Kcal

What time did you eat?

Breakfas: .... Lunch: .... Dinner: .... Snack 1: .... Snack 2: ....

Supplements/............

Sports activities

Bad habits:
Cigarettes
Alcohol
Sweets
Coffee

How do you feel today?

Other: ....

Notes of the day

Week 8

This week we focus on condiments that often go into the background because they are not always so visible (think of salt, vinegar, or oil) but they hinder our well-being.

The condiments can be divided into five categories:

Vegetable oils - extra virgin olive oil, linseed, sesame, sunflower, peanut oil
Vinegar and citrus juices - apple vinegar, wine, citrus juice...
Spices and herbs - salt, pepper, oregano, thyme, rosemary, curry...
Animal fat - butter, cream
Gastronomic sauces - mayonnaise, mustard, ketchup

As we saw two weeks ago, vegetable oils, spices and herbs are foods rich in unsaturated fats that are good for our body if consumed in small quantities; too elaborate condiments, such as gastronomic sauces or derived from animals, contribute to raising blood cholesterol levels and expose us to different diseases.

Salt is the spice we are most fond of but, in addition to influencing swelling and water retention, it increases our blood pressure: there are at least seven healthier foods that can replace the salt on the table, let's see them together.

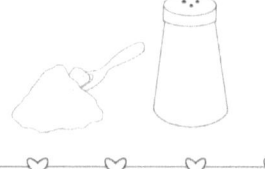

- The aromatic bouquet can be made up of the herbs we prefer, but the most suitable to replace the coarse salt in the pasta are celery, fennel, thyme, parsley, and marjoram. To flavor the water, we can put the ingredients in a bag of tulle and leave it to soak until cooked;

- The celery salt is used in Bloody Mary and consists simply of dried or baked celery stalks;

- Inactive food yeast is the infamous seasoning agent of vegans who use it instead of cheese: it is made from brewer's yeast and is found in organic supermarkets;

- Soy sauce can be used in cooking to caramelize second courses or vegetables or as an alternative dressing for salad;

- Lemon juice is another excellent dressing for salads and can be combined with vinegar, mustard, yoghurt, honey, spices and herbs to our liking;

- Miso comes from the fermentation of soya beans and from cereals such as rice and barley. Its flavor is so strong that it can be used instead of the kitchen nut.

- Gomasio is ideal for dressing salads, soups and velvety. It is a condiment native to Japan and we can recreate it at home using whole sea salt together with roasted sesame seeds.

Challenge of the week:

FIND A WAY TO REPLACE SALT ON THREE DIFFERENT DAYS DURING THIS WEEK AND LIMIT ITS USE TO THE KITCHEN (DO NOT BRING IT TO THE TABLE). SOON YOU'LL BE ABLE TO STICK IT AT THE BOTTOM OF THE SPICE CABINET AND FORGET ABOUT IT!

Days 50   Date ....../ ....../ ......

Breakfast   Lunch   Dinner

Snack 1   Snack 2

🥤 Water

🛏 Sleep

🍽 Kcal

What time did you eat?

Breakfas: .... Lunch: .... Dinner: .... Snack 1: .... Snack 2: ....

Supplements/ ....   Sports activities

Bad habits:
Cigarettes
Alcohol
Sweets
Coffee

How do you feel today?

Other: ....

Notes of the day

Days 51   Date ....../ ....../ ......

Breakfast   Lunch   Dinner

Snack 1   Snack 2   Water

Sleep

Kcal

What time did you eat?

Breakfas: .... Lunch: .... Dinner: .... Snack 1: .... Snack 2: ....

Supplements/ ....   Sports activities

Bad habits: How do you feel today?
Cigarettes
Alcohol
Sweets
Coffee   Other: ....

Notes of the day

Days ♡52♡   Date ....../ ....../ ......

Breakfast   Lunch   Dinner

Snack 1   Snack 2   🥛 Water

🛏 Sleep

🍽 Kcal

What time did you eat?

Breakfas: .... Lunch: .... Dinner: .... Snack 1: .... Snack 2: ....

Supplements/ ....

Sports activities

Bad habits:
Cigarettes
Alcohol
Sweets
Coffee

How do you feel today?

☺ ☹ 😐 😣 😴

Other: ....

Notes of the day

Days 53   Date ....../....../......

Breakfast   Lunch   Dinner

Snack 1   Snack 2

 Water

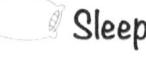 Sleep

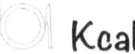 Kcal

What time did you eat?

Breakfas: .... Lunch: .... Dinner: .... Snack 1: .... Snack 2: ....

Supplements/............   Sports activities

Bad habits: How do you feel today?
Cigarettes
Alcohol
Sweets
Coffee   Other: ....

Notes of the day

Days 54   Date ....../ ....../ ......

Breakfast

Lunch

Dinner

Snack 1

Snack 2

 Water

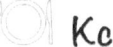 Sleep

Kcal

What time did you eat?

Breakfas: ....   Lunch: ....   Dinner: ....   Snack 1: ....   Snack 2: ....

Supplements/ ....

Sports activities

Bad habits:
Cigarettes
Alcohol
Sweets
Coffee

How do you feel today?

Other: ....

Notes of the day

Days ♡55♡   Date ....../ ....../ ......

Breakfast   Lunch   Dinner

Snack 1   Snack 2   ☐ Water

☐ Sleep

☐ Kcal

What time did you eat?

Breakfas: .... Lunch: .... Dinner: .... Snack 1: .... Snack 2: ....

Supplements/ ....

Sports activities

Bad habits:
Cigarettes
Alcohol
Sweets
Coffee

How do you feel today?

☺ ☹ 😐 😠 😴

Other: ....

Notes of the day

Days ♡56♡　　Date ....../ ....../ ......

Breakfast　　Lunch　　Dinner

Snack 1　　Snack 2　　🥛 Water

🫓 Sleep

🍽 Kcal

What time did you eat?

Breakfas: .... Lunch: .... Dinner: .... Snack 1: .... Snack 2: ....

Supplements/ ....　　♡　Sports activities

Bad habits:
Cigarettes
Alcohol
Sweets
Coffee

How do you feel today?

🙂　🙁　😐　😣　😴

Other: ....

Notes of the day

Week 9

This week we're talking about colors. I know, I'm accompanying you on a food journey to educate you to eat the right way and not to do a session of Seasonal Color Analysis, but colors are everywhere and, often, we don't give them the right importance.

Every day we should eat at least five servings of fruit and vegetables, understood as two of vegetables and three of fruit, so as to keep us healthy. In addition to this, we should also vary the color of the foods we consume to ensure that we take on all their nutritional properties.

Below, let's see which foods correspond to the various colors of the rainbow and that must never be missing on the table:

blue/purple - aubergines, figs, raspberries, blueberries, black grapes, blackberries, blackcurrants, plums, radicchio contain potassium, magnesium, vitamin C and beta carotene;

green - asparagus, rocket, parsley, spinach, white grapes, kiwi, zucchini, salad, artichokes, cucumbers, broccoli, basil contain beta carotene, folic acid, vitamin C and magnesium;

white - bananas, cauliflower, garlic, onions, fennel, mushrooms, pears, apples, leeks contain vitamin C, potassium, polyphenols, selenium and sulfur compounds;

yellow - oranges, mandarins, lemons, melons, apricots, fish, carrots, peppers, pumpkin are rich in potassium, beta carotene, flavonoids and vitamin C.

orange/red - watermelons, red oranges, cherries, strawberries, peppers, radishes, tomatoes contain anthocyanins and lycopene.

Challenge of the week:

THIS WEEK MAKE SURE YOU EAT ALL THESE COLORS THROUGHOUT THE DAY FOR AT LEAST ONE MEAL EACH DAY.

Days ♡57♡

Date ....../ ....../ ......

Breakfast

Lunch

Dinner

Snack 1

Snack 2

Water

Sleep

Kcal

What time did you eat?

Breakfas: .... Lunch: .... Dinner: .... Snack 1: .... Snack 2: ....

Supplements/ ....

Sports activities

Bad habits:
Cigarettes
Alcohol
Sweets
Coffee

How do you feel today?

☺ ☹ 😐 😠 😴

Other: ....

Notes of the day

Days 58   Date ....../ ....../ ......

Breakfast   Lunch   Dinner

Snack 1   Snack 2

 Water

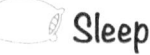 Sleep

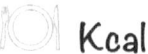 Kcal

What time did you eat?

Breakfas: .... Lunch: .... Dinner: .... Snack 1: .... Snack 2: ....

Supplements/............

Sports activities

Bad habits:
Cigarettes
Alcohol
Sweets
Coffee

How do you feel today?

Other: ....

Notes of the day

Days ♡59♡

Date ....../ ....../ ......

Breakfast

Lunch

Dinner

Snack 1

Snack 2

 Water

 Sleep

 Kcal

What time did you eat?

Breakfas: .... Lunch: .... Dinner: .... Snack 1: .... Snack 2: ....

Supplements/ ....

Sports activities

Bad habits:
Cigarettes
Alcohol
Sweets
Coffee

How do you feel today?

Other: ....

Notes of the day

Days 60

Date ....../ ....../ ......

Breakfast

Lunch

Dinner

Snack 1

Snack 2

Water

Sleep

Kcal

What time did you eat?

Breakfas: ....   Lunch: ....   Dinner: ....   Snack 1: ....   Snack 2: ....

Supplements/ ....

Sports activities

Bad habits:
Cigarettes
Alcohol
Sweets
Coffee

How do you feel today?

☺ ☹ 😐 😠 😴

Other: ....

Notes of the day

How was your second month?

Let's get back in shape!

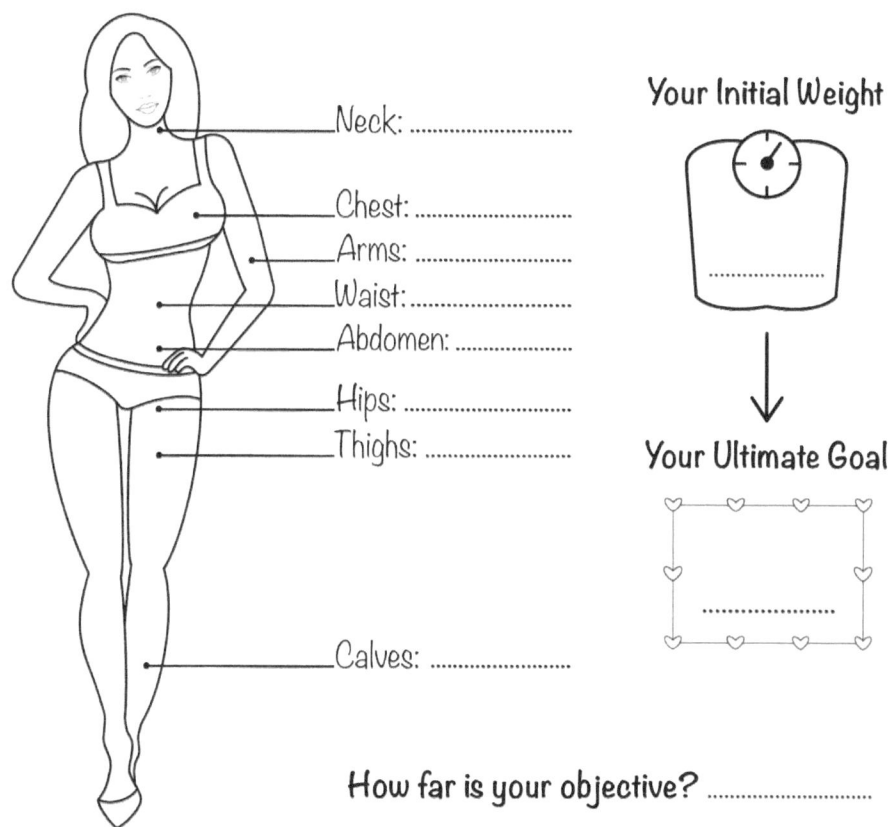

Neck: ....

Chest: ....

Arms: ....

Waist: ....

Abdomen: ....

Hips: ....

Thighs: ....

Calves: ....

Your Initial Weight

....

Your Ultimate Goal

....

How far is your objective? ....

Write your thoughts about these weeks!

Days ♡61♡

Date ....../ ....../ ......

Breakfast   Lunch   Dinner

Snack 1   Snack 2

☐ Water

☐ Sleep

☐ Kcal

What time did you eat?

Breakfas: .... Lunch: .... Dinner: .... Snack 1: .... Snack 2: ....

Supplements/ ....   ♡ Sports activities

Bad habits: ♡ How do you feel today?
Cigarettes
Alcohol   ☺ ☹ 😐 😠 😴
Sweets
Coffee   Other: ....

Notes of the day

Days ♡62♡   Date ....../ ....../ ......

Breakfast   Lunch   Dinner

Snack 1   Snack 2

🥛 Water

🛏 Sleep

🍽 Kcal

What time did you eat?

Breakfas: ....   Lunch: ....   Dinner: ....   Snack 1: ....   Snack 2: ....

Supplements/ ....   ♡ Sports activities

Bad habits: How do you feel today?
Cigarettes
Alcohol   😊 🙁 😐 😠 😴
Sweets
Coffee   Other: ....

Notes of the day

Days (63)   Date ....../ ....../ ......

Breakfast   Lunch   Dinner

Snack 1   Snack 2

 Water

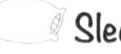 Sleep

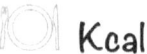 Kcal

What time did you eat?

Breakfas: .... Lunch: .... Dinner: .... Snack 1: .... Snack 2: ....

Supplements/ ....   Sports activities

Bad habits: How do you feel today?
Cigarettes
Alcohol
Sweets
Coffee   Other: ....

Notes of the day

Week 10

If you, too, walked past the milk rack at the supermarket and wondered at least once **how they make vegetable milk**, this week I will light you up and probably let you out of your comfort zone of animal milk.

We have always drunk cow's milk, since we were little, probably because at the time there was not much variety as today, and now we continue to buy that milk more out of habit than by choice, you see yourself in this situation?

Vegetable milk undergoes a process that transforms soya, almonds, oats and other vegetable products into a dense paste or flour that is diluted with water and to which vitamins and minerals are added.

The substantial difference between vegetable and animal milk is that the former contains less carbohydrates, less harmful fats and more good fats, while the latter naturally contains vitamin D and calcium.
The most common types of vegetable milk are three: almond milk, soy milk and oat milk.

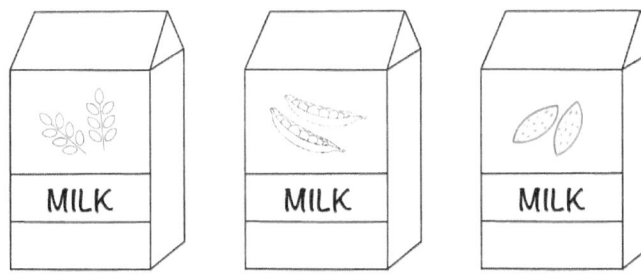

- Almond and oat milk have very little protein compared to cow's milk, but the milk that contains the least nutrients is almond milk.

- Oat milk is rich in betaglucans, a type of fiber that is good for our health and contains carbohydrates, sometimes as much as cow's milk.

- Soya milk has as much protein as cow's milk and is rich in potassium. It is not a race, there is no winning milk and one worse of all: the choice of milk depends on our needs, on our allergies or intolerances, but all the types of milk we have available offer enough nutrients to be part of a healthy and balanced diet.

As you may have guessed, this week's focus is to make a conscious choice and not bring guided by inertia every time you buy milk at the supermarket.

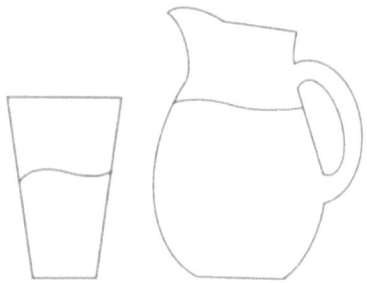

Challenge of the week:
GET OUT OF YOUR COMFORT ZONE AND BUY A BRICK OF ALL KINDS OF VEGETABLE MILK THAT INSPIRES YOU MOST AT THE SUPERMARKET AND REPLACE COW'S MILK FOR AT LEAST THREE DAYS THIS WEEK.

Days ♡64♡　　　Date ....../ ....../ ......

Breakfast　　Lunch　　Dinner

Snack 1　　Snack 2　　🥛 Water

🍋 Sleep

🍽 Kcal

What time did you eat?

Breakfas: ....　Lunch: ....　Dinner: ....　Snack 1: ....　Snack 2: ....

Supplements/ ....　♡ Sports activities

Bad habits:　　♡ How do you feel today?
Cigarettes
Alcohol　　　　😊　😞　😐　😖　😴
Sweets
Coffee　　　　Other: ....

Notes of the day

Days ♡65♡

Date ....../....../......

Breakfast

Lunch

Dinner

Snack 1

Snack 2

Water

Sleep

Kcal

What time did you eat?

Breakfas: .... Lunch: .... Dinner: .... Snack 1: .... Snack 2: ....

Supplements/............

Sports activities

Bad habits:
Cigarettes
Alcohol
Sweets
Coffee

How do you feel today?

☺ ☹ 😐 😠 😴

Other: ....

Notes of the day

Days ♡66♡

Date ....../ ....../ ......

Breakfast

Lunch

Dinner

Snack 1

Snack 2

🥛 Water

🛏 Sleep

🍽 Kcal

What time did you eat?

Breakfas: .... Lunch: .... Dinner: .... Snack 1: .... Snack 2: ....

Supplements/............

Sports activities

Bad habits:
Cigarettes
Alcohol
Sweets
Coffee

How do you feel today?

☺ ☹ 😐 😣 😴

Other: ....

Notes of the day

Days 67   Date ....../ ....../ ......

Breakfast   Lunch   Dinner

Snack I   Snack 2   Water

Sleep

Kcal

What time did you eat?

Breakfas: .... Lunch: .... Dinner: .... Snack I: .... Snack 2: ....

Supplements/ ....   Sports activities

Bad habits: How do you feel today?
Cigarettes
Alcohol   ☺ ☹ 😐 😠 😴
Sweets
Coffee   Other: ....

Notes of the day

Days 68

Date ....../ ....../ ......

Breakfast

Lunch

Dinner

Snack 1

Snack 2

 Water

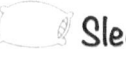 Sleep

 Kcal

What time did you eat?

Breakfas: .... Lunch: .... Dinner: .... Snack 1: .... Snack 2: ....

Supplements/ ....

Sports activities

Bad habits:
Cigarettes
Alcohol
Sweets
Coffee

How do you feel today?

Other: ....

Notes of the day

Days ♡69♡ Date ....../ ....../ ......

Breakfast

Lunch

Dinner

Snack 1

Snack 2

 Water

 Sleep

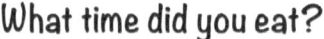 Kcal

What time did you eat?

Breakfas: .... Lunch: .... Dinner: .... Snack 1: .... Snack 2: ....

Supplements/ ....

Sports activities

Bad habits:
Cigarettes
Alcohol
Sweets
Coffee

How do you feel today?

Other: ....

Notes of the day

Days ♡70♡

Date ....../ ....../ ......

Breakfast

Lunch

Dinner

Snack 1

Snack 2

Water

Sleep

Kcal

What time did you eat?

Breakfas: .... Lunch: .... Dinner: .... Snack 1: .... Snack 2: ....

Supplements/ ....

Sports activities

Bad habits:
Cigarettes
Alcohol
Sweets
Coffee

How do you feel today?

☺ ☹ 😐 😣 😴

Other: ....

Notes of the day

Week 11

If you're trying to eat healthier, the best thing to do is to make sure that you always have something ready at hand, so you don't fall into temptation.

Below, you will find some tips to prepare everything you need in advance and always have something available: the only ingredient you will have to add will be a pinch of creativity! Let's get started right away.

1. Prepare the cereals and legumes: chickpeas, lentils, brown rice, quinoa must be soaked in water for about 12 hours before cooking, to make them more digestible (even only 2 hours make the difference!). Once ready, rinse well and cook them following the instructions. You can decide to keep half a portion in the fridge and to freeze the other half;

2. Prepare the vegetables: to eat them fresh during the week, you can cut and store them in a bowl full of water that will also keep them crisp;

3. Prepare the bread: cut the durum wheat bread into slices so as to freeze it already cut and thaw only the amount of bread that will serve you;

4. Prepare the vegetables to be baked in the oven: sweet potatoes, Roman cabbage, broccoli, pumpkin, eggplant... you can cook in advance the vegetables you will eat during the week and keep half in the fridge and half in the freezer, so that you have them available for several days;

5. You can use a portion of cooked chickpeas to make hummus, while with cooked eggplants you can create an alternative dressing for salads and babaganoush, a sauce very similar to hummus;

6. For breakfast, you can prepare in advance a banana bread or a yogurt plumcake that can be cut and frozen just like bread, and you can also store fruit in the freezer, so that you always have it on hand without the risk of it going bad.

The advantage of preparing ingredients in advance for use during the week, as well as always having something healthy available and not having to resort to takeaway or industrial foods, it's a big time saver and we won't have to despair to run to the supermarket several times a week.

Having a shopping list always up to date is the secret not to be tempted among the departments of the supermarket: you can decide to have it printed in the old-fashioned way or to have it in the notes of your phone, to keep it always at hand!

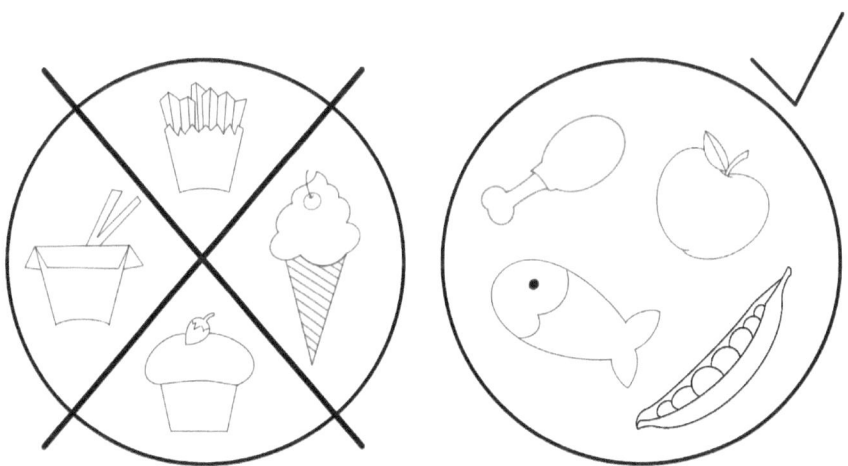

Challenge of the week:
TAKE A DAY WHEN YOU ORGANIZE THE SHOPPING LIST AND, AFTER BUYING ALL THE INGREDIENTS, PUT YOURSELF AT THE STOVE AND COOK TO BE SURE TO HAVE EVERYTHING READY FOR AT LEAST SEVEN DAYS. THE SECRET IS TO CUT IN ADVANCE AND FREEZE!

Days ♡ 71

Date ....../ ....../ ......

Breakfast   Lunch   Dinner

Snack 1   Snack 2

□ Water

▱ Sleep

🍽 Kcal

What time did you eat?

Breakfas: .... Lunch: .... Dinner: .... Snack 1: .... Snack 2: ....

Supplements/ ....   Sports activities

Bad habits: How do you feel today?
Cigarettes
Alcohol   ☺ ☹ 😐 😠 😴
Sweets
Coffee   Other: ....

Notes of the day

Days ♡72♡   Date ....../ ....../ ......

Breakfast   Lunch   Dinner

Snack 1   Snack 2

 Water

 Sleep

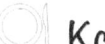 Kcal

What time did you eat?

Breakfas: .... Lunch: .... Dinner: .... Snack 1: .... Snack 2: ....

Supplements/ ....   Sports activities

Bad habits:
Cigarettes   How do you feel today?
Alcohol
Sweets
Coffee
              Other: ....

Notes of the day

Days ♡73♡

Date ....../ ....../ ......

Breakfast   ## Lunch   ## Dinner

Snack 1   ## Snack 2

 Water

 Sleep

Kcal

What time did you eat?

Breakfas: .... Lunch: .... Dinner: .... Snack 1: .... Snack 2: ....

Supplements/ ....   Sports activities

Bad habits: How do you feel today?
Cigarettes
Alcohol
Sweets
Coffee   Other: ....

Notes of the day

Days 74

Date ....../ ....../ ......

Breakfast

Lunch

Dinner

Snack 1

Snack 2

 Water

Sleep

Kcal

What time did you eat?

Breakfas: .... Lunch: .... Dinner: .... Snack 1: .... Snack 2: ....

Supplements/ ....

Sports activities

Bad habits:
Cigarettes
Alcohol
Sweets
Coffee

How do you feel today?

Other: ....

Notes of the day

Days 75   Date ....../ ....../ ......

Breakfast   Lunch   Dinner

Snack 1   Snack 2   Water

Sleep

Kcal

What time did you eat?

Breakfas: ....   Lunch: ....   Dinner: ....   Snack 1: ....   Snack 2: ....

Supplements/ ....   Sports activities

Bad habits: How do you feel today?
Cigarettes
Alcohol
Sweets
Coffee

Other: ....

Notes of the day

In these seventy-five days

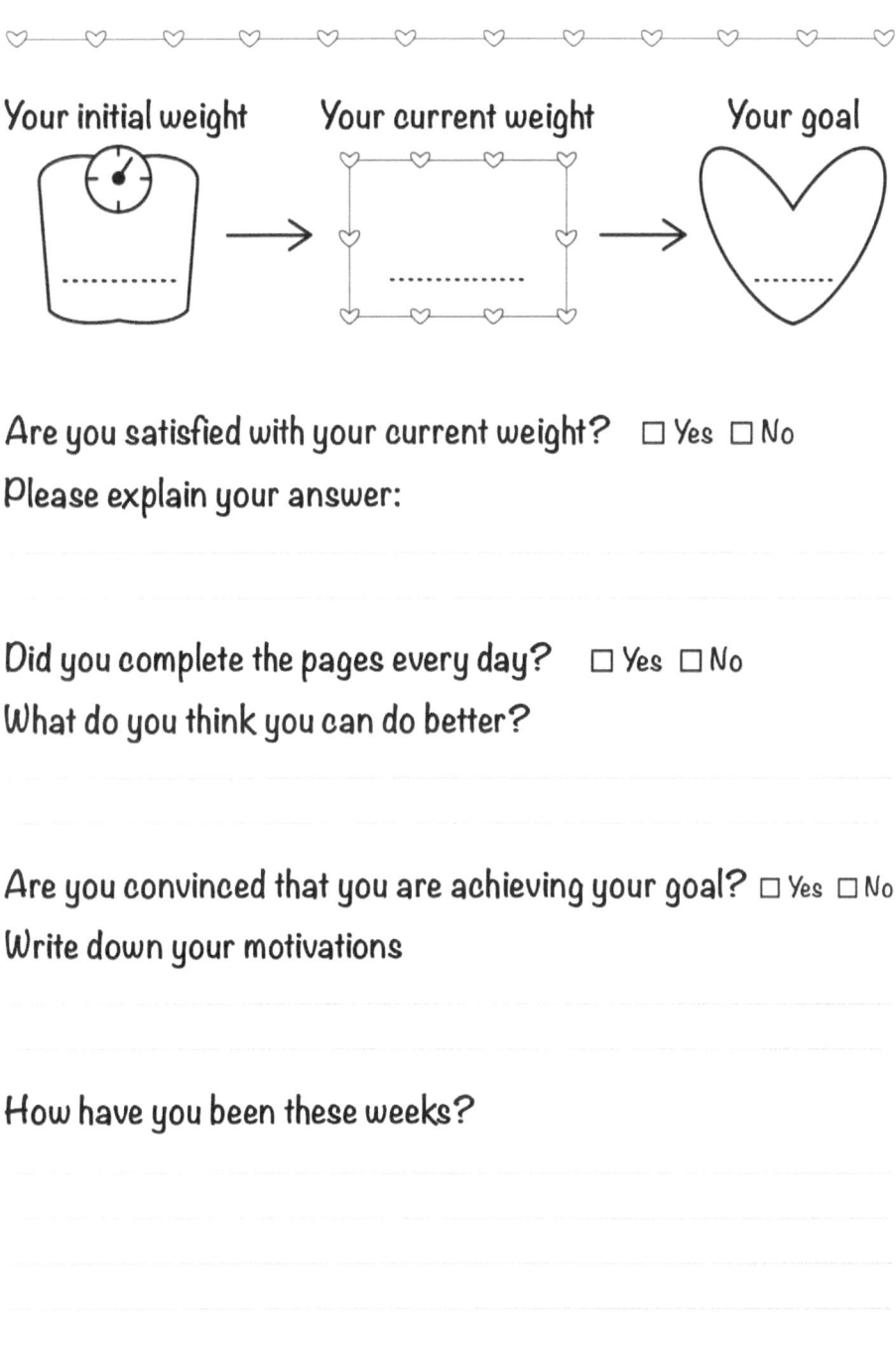

Your initial weight   Your current weight   Your goal

Are you satisfied with your current weight?   ☐ Yes ☐ No
Please explain your answer:

Did you complete the pages every day?   ☐ Yes ☐ No
What do you think you can do better?

Are you convinced that you are achieving your goal? ☐ Yes ☐ No
Write down your motivations

How have you been these weeks?

Days 76 Date ....../ ....../ ......

Breakfast　　Lunch　　Dinner

Snack 1　　Snack 2

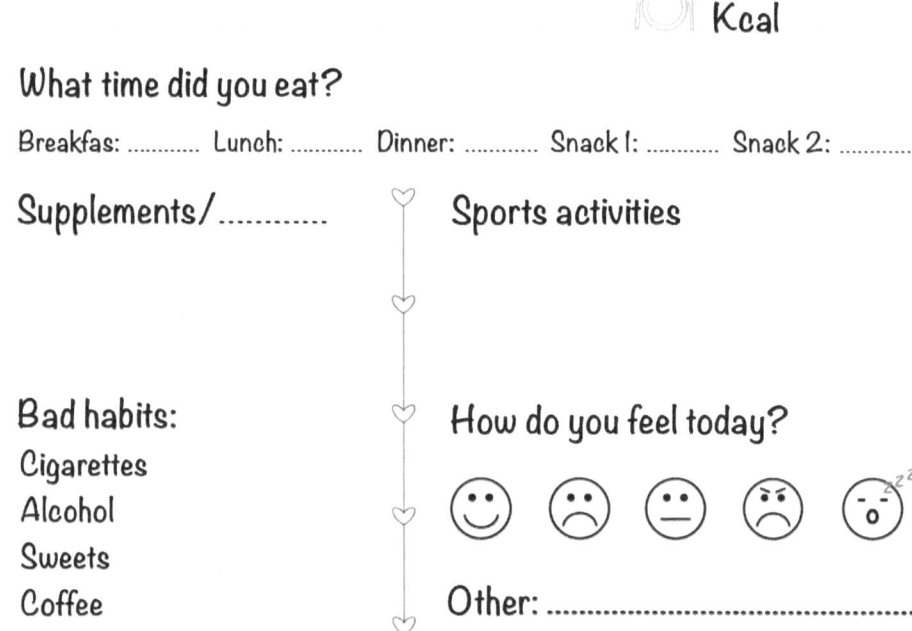

Water

Sleep

Kcal

What time did you eat?

Breakfas: ....　Lunch: ....　Dinner: ....　Snack 1: ....　Snack 2: ....

Supplements/ ....

Sports activities

Bad habits:
Cigarettes
Alcohol
Sweets
Coffee

How do you feel today?

Other: ....

Notes of the day

Days ♡ 77   Date ....../ ....../ ......

Breakfast   Lunch   Dinner

Snack 1   Snack 2

Water

Sleep

Kcal

What time did you eat?

Breakfas: .... Lunch: .... Dinner: .... Snack 1: .... Snack 2: ....

Supplements/ ....   Sports activities

Bad habits:
Cigarettes
Alcohol
Sweets
Coffee

How do you feel today?

Other: ....

Notes of the day

Week 12

You didn't hear the alarm or, better, you heard it, but you decided to ignore it and sleep for 5 minutes more that have become 30 in the blink of an eye, you have little time to prepare and even less to eat a bite before you run to work: is this a scenario that has already been seen time and time again?

Unfortunately, the morning is not for everyone: you can't force an owl to be perky when the sun rises, as you can't force a lark to stay up late. Each of us has its own rhythms and not everyone is happy to set the alarm clock an hour early in the morning to do things calmly or go for a ride. There is no doubt, however, that we can all be organized and not be reduced to the last second to prepare, especially when we have schedules to respect.

Breakfast is the most important meal of the day: how many times have we been told? And yet...
With breakfast we already ensure 20/30% of the caloric intake we need every day and so, skipping it, we will not have the energy to start the day at best but, on the contrary, we will have difficulty concentrating and we will not be vigilant enough or reactive.

Skipping breakfast means putting our bodies in a fast situation from dinner the night before until lunch and, as a result, we will need to fill that rumble in the stomach with something ready and quick to consume, like snacks at vending machines.
To avoid falling into this trap, we can anticipate and prepare a take-out breakfast to take to work, such as a yogurt with fresh fruit, a teaspoon of peanut butter and granola.

The ideal would be to be able to have breakfast calmly at home, perhaps preparing the table the evening before going to sleep and consume proteins (present in milk or its derivatives) that regulate our glycemic index, cereals and fruits that provide the correct carbohydrate, fiber and sugar intake.

Below, you will find suggestions to integrate breakfast and soon you will realize that you can no longer do without:

1. Never skip it - breakfast is as necessary a meal as lunch and dinner;
2. Never less than 15 minutes - throughout the day we are used to running so as not to arrive late to the thousand commitments that await us: let's enjoy this meal in peace;
3. Drinking coffee at the bar in a hurry does not mean having breakfast - it is a meal and, as such, you have to eat something, not just drink;
4. Fruit - a juice or seasonal fruit should never be missing on the table next to biscuits, wholemeal bread, rusks, cereals and yogurt;
5. Varieties - try to vary each day by adding a new ingredient or alternating your favorites.
6. Take time - to buy time, you can prepare the table the night before (and the excuse of not having time no longer holds!);
7. Set a good example - if your boys see you skipping breakfast, it will be difficult for them not to get into the same habit.

Challenge of the week:
MAKE SURE YOU HAVE A HEALTHY AND BALANCED BREAKFAST AT HOME OR TAKE AWAY AT LEAST THREE DAYS THIS WEEK.

Days ♡78♡   Date ....../ ....../ ......

Breakfast   Lunch   Dinner

Snack 1   Snack 2   Water

Sleep

Kcal

What time did you eat?

Breakfas: .... Lunch: .... Dinner: .... Snack 1: .... Snack 2: ....

Supplements/ ....   ♡   **Sports activities**

Bad habits: **How do you feel today?**
Cigarettes
Alcohol   ☺ ☹ 😐 😠 😴
Sweets
Coffee   Other: ....

Notes of the day

Days 79

Date ....../ ....../ ......

Breakfast

Lunch

Dinner

Snack 1

Snack 2

Water

Sleep

Kcal

What time did you eat?

Breakfas: .... Lunch: .... Dinner: .... Snack 1: .... Snack 2: ....

Supplements/ ....

Sports activities

Bad habits:
Cigarettes
Alcohol
Sweets
Coffee

How do you feel today?

Other: ....

Notes of the day

Days 80   Date ....../ ....../ ......

Breakfast   Lunch   Dinner

Snack 1   Snack 2

 Water

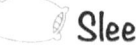 Sleep

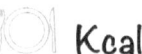 Kcal

What time did you eat?

Breakfas: .... Lunch: .... Dinner: .... Snack 1: .... Snack 2: ....

Supplements/ ....   Sports activities

Bad habits: How do you feel today?
Cigarettes
Alcohol
Sweets
Coffee

Other: ....

Notes of the day

Days ♡81♡

Date ....../ ....../ ......

Breakfast

Lunch

Dinner

Snack 1

Snack 2

 Water

Sleep

Kcal

What time did you eat?

Breakfas: .... Lunch: .... Dinner: .... Snack 1: .... Snack 2: ....

Supplements/ ....

Sports activities

Bad habits:
Cigarettes
Alcohol
Sweets
Coffee

How do you feel today?

Other: ....

Notes of the day

Days ♡82♡   Date ....../ ....../ ......

Breakfast   ## Lunch   ## Dinner

Snack 1   ## Snack 2   Water

Sleep

Kcal

What time did you eat?

Breakfas: .... Lunch: .... Dinner: .... Snack 1: .... Snack 2: ....

Supplements/ ....   Sports activities

Bad habits: How do you feel today?
Cigarettes
Alcohol   ☺ ☹ 😐 😠 😴
Sweets
Coffee   Other: ....

Notes of the day

Days ♡83♡   Date ....../ ....../ ......

Breakfast   ## Lunch   ## Dinner

Snack 1   ## Snack 2   Water

Sleep

Kcal

What time did you eat?

Breakfas: .... Lunch: .... Dinner: .... Snack 1: .... Snack 2: ....

Supplements/ ....   ♡   Sports activities

Bad habits: How do you feel today?
Cigarettes
Alcohol
Sweets
Coffee   Other: ....

Notes of the day

Days ♡84♡

Date ..../......./......

Breakfast

Lunch

Dinner

Snack 1

Snack 2

Water

Sleep

Kcal

What time did you eat?

Breakfas: .... Lunch: .... Dinner: .... Snack 1: .... Snack 2: ....

Supplements/ ....

Sports activities

Bad habits:
Cigarettes
Alcohol
Sweets
Coffee

How do you feel today?

☺ ☹ 😐 😠 😴

Other: ....

Notes of the day

Week 13

The key word of this last week is **movement**: I know, you might shiver at this word and the idea of getting off the couch after eight hours of work is not tempting. I'll tell you a secret: we are beings made of mental and physical energy that needs to be moved in some way.
We can't think of wasting our lives sitting around all day, between the office chair, the couch and the car seat.

Getting around and doing physical activity is essential to ensure our psychophysical well-being, but this does not mean forcing us to set the alarm an hour before for the canonical morning run or enroll in the gym and then never find the desire or time to go.
Physical activity is everywhere: we can take the journey from the car to the office to take a quick walk, we can take the lunch break to do a yoga session at home or outdoors, we can choose to take the stairs instead of the elevator...

The choices we make every day determine our physical and mental well-being because moving allows us to keep our metabolism alive, allows us to refine the capacity of our alveoli, to allow us to have more breath even with the advancing age, improves blood circulation and our musculoskeletal system.
In addition to all these physical advantages, physical activity allows us to fight the stress and tensions accumulated during the day, thanks to the endorphins it releases.

Challenge of the week:

TRY TO DEDICATE AT LEAST 20/30 MINUTES A DAY TO PHYSICAL ACTIVITY OF **ANY KIND**: FROM MORNING RUNNING, TO FAST WALKING OR A SIMPLE WALK IN NATURE OR IN THE SHOPS, STRETCHING TO YOGA. ANY CHOSEN ACTIVITY IS FINE, IT DOESN'T HAVE TO BE TOO INTENSE IF YOU'RE NOT USED TO MOVING. LISTEN TO YOUR BODY.

P.S. Dancing to the rhythm of your teenage songs is also considered movement, so it applies!

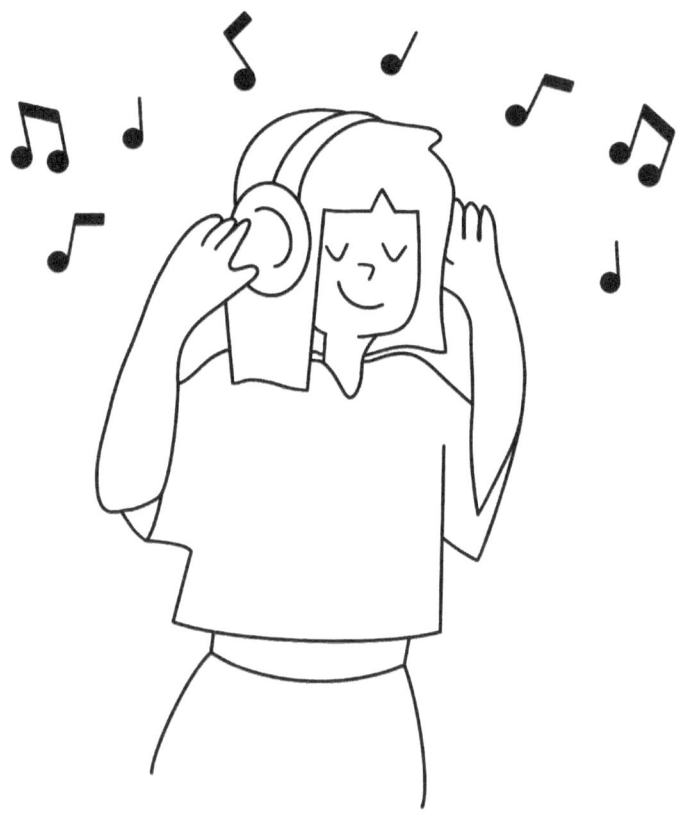

Days 85   Date ....../....../......

Breakfast   Lunch   Dinner

Snack 1   Snack 2   Water

 Sleep

Kcal

What time did you eat?

Breakfas: ....   Lunch: ....   Dinner: ....   Snack 1: ....   Snack 2: ....

Supplements/ ....   Sports activities

Bad habits: How do you feel today?
Cigarettes
Alcohol
Sweets
Coffee   Other: ....

Notes of the day

Days 86

Date ....../ ....../ ......

Breakfast

Lunch

Dinner

Snack 1

Snack 2

Water

Sleep

Kcal

What time did you eat?

Breakfas: .... Lunch: .... Dinner: .... Snack 1: .... Snack 2: ....

Supplements/ ....

Sports activities

Bad habits:
Cigarettes
Alcohol
Sweets
Coffee

How do you feel today?

:) :(:| :((zzz)

Other: ....

Notes of the day

Days ♡87♡

Date ....../ ....../ ......

Breakfast   Lunch   Dinner

Snack 1   Snack 2

Water

Sleep

Kcal

What time did you eat?

Breakfas: ....   Lunch: ....   Dinner: ....   Snack 1: ....   Snack 2: ....

Supplements/ ....

Sports activities

Bad habits:
Cigarettes
Alcohol
Sweets
Coffee

How do you feel today?

☺   ☹   😐   😠   😴

Other: ....

Notes of the day

Days ♡88♡

Date ....../ ....../ ......

Breakfast   Lunch   Dinner

Snack 1   Snack 2

Water

Sleep

Kcal

What time did you eat?

Breakfas: .... Lunch: .... Dinner: .... Snack 1: .... Snack 2: ....

Supplements/ ....   Sports activities

Bad habits:
Cigarettes
Alcohol
Sweets
Coffee

How do you feel today?

☺ ☹ 😐 😠 😴

Other: ....

Notes of the day

Days 89   Date ....../ ....../ ......

Breakfast   Lunch   Dinner

Snack 1   Snack 2   Water
                                     Sleep
                                     Kcal

What time did you eat?

Breakfas: .... Lunch: .... Dinner: .... Snack 1: .... Snack 2: ....

Supplements/ ....   Sports activities

Bad habits: How do you feel today?
Cigarettes
Alcohol   :) :(:| >:((-_-)zz
Sweets
Coffee   Other: ....

Notes of the day

Days ♡90♡

Date ....../ ....../ ......

Breakfast   Lunch   Dinner

Snack 1   Snack 2

🥛 Water

🛏 Sleep

🍽 Kcal

What time did you eat?

Breakfas: .... Lunch: .... Dinner: .... Snack 1: .... Snack 2: ....

Supplements/ ....

Sports activities

Bad habits:
Cigarettes
Alcohol
Sweets
Coffee

How do you feel today?

☺ ☹ 😐 😠 😴

Other: ....

Notes of the day

How was your third month?

Let's get back in shape!

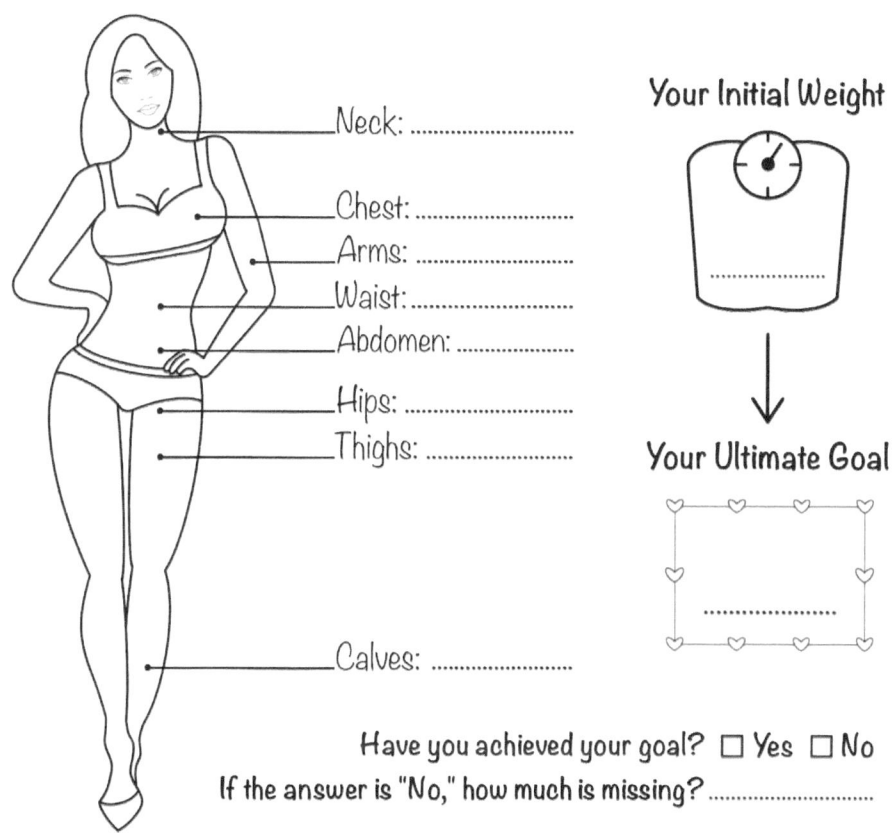

Neck: ....

Chest: ....

Arms: ....

Waist: ....

Abdomen: ....

Hips: ....

Thighs: ....

Calves: ....

Your Initial Weight

....

Your Ultimate Goal

....

Have you achieved your goal? ☐ Yes ☐ No

If the answer is "No," how much is missing? ....

Write your thoughts about these weeks!

Shoot and paste your final photo

Front

Shoot and paste your final photo

Back

Notes

Notes

Notes

Here you are! Congratulations on coming to the end, being here is already a great victory!

Don't worry if you haven't achieved the result you expected, you can always continue this journey with us by buying another diary and go on until you reach the goal!

Finally, answer these questions for a complete overview of your experience!

Are you happy with the final result? ☐ Yes ☐ No
Give reasons for your answer!

Did you find this book useful? Why?

What do you think you need to improve?

Which initial goals have you achieved? ☐ 1 ☐ 2 ☐ 3
Mark them with a cross

Thank you!

www.ingramcontent.com/pod-product-compliance
Lightning Source LLC
Chambersburg PA
CBHW020249290526
45784CB00003B/1168